Clean & Lean
PREGNANCY GUIDE

James Duigan

with Maria Lally

Photography by
Sebastian Roos and Charlie Richards

Kyle Books

First published in Great Britain in 2014 by
Kyle Books, an imprint of Kyle Cathie Ltd
192–198 Vauxhall Bridge Road
London SW1V 1DX
www.kylebooks.com

10 9 8 7 6 5 4 3 2 1
ISBN 978-0-85783-105-7

Text © 2014 James Duigan and Maria Lally
Design © 2014 Kyle Books
Location photographs © 2014 Sebastian Roos
Recipe and food photographs © 2014 Charlie Richards
p. 7 © Angelo Pennetta / Trunk Archive, p. 16 © David Gubert / Chilli Media,
p. 21 © Pierre Toussaint, p. 103 © Holly Valance

Project Editor: Judith Hannam
Copy Editor: Anne Newman
Designer: Dale Walker
Model: Christiane Duigan
Recipe Home Economy: Mima Sinclair
Recipe Styling: Olivia Wardle
Production: Nic Jones, David Hearn and Lisa Pinnell

A Cataloguing in Publication record for this title is available from the British Library.

Colour reproduction by ALTA, London
Printed and bound in China by C & C Offset Printing Co., Ltd

The information and advice contained in this book are intended as a general guide.
Neither the author nor the publishers can be held responsible for claims arising from
the inappropriate use of any remedy or exercise regime. Do not attempt self-
diagnosis or self-treatment for serious or long-term conditions before consulting a
medical professional or qualified practitioner. Do not begin any exercise programme
or undertake any self-treatment while taking other prescribed drugs or receiving
therapy without first seeking professional guidance. Always seek medical advice if
any symptoms persist.

Clean & Lean
PREGNANCY
GUIDE

THE HEALTHY WAY TO EXERCISE AND EAT
BEFORE, DURING AND AFTER PREGNANCY

James Duigan

James Duigan, world-renowned wellness guru and owner of Bodyism, London's premier health and fitness facility, is one of the world's top personal trainers. Bodyism's glittering client list includes Rosie Huntington-Whiteley, Lara Stone, David Gandy, Holly Valance and Hugh Grant.

9030 00004 1563 2

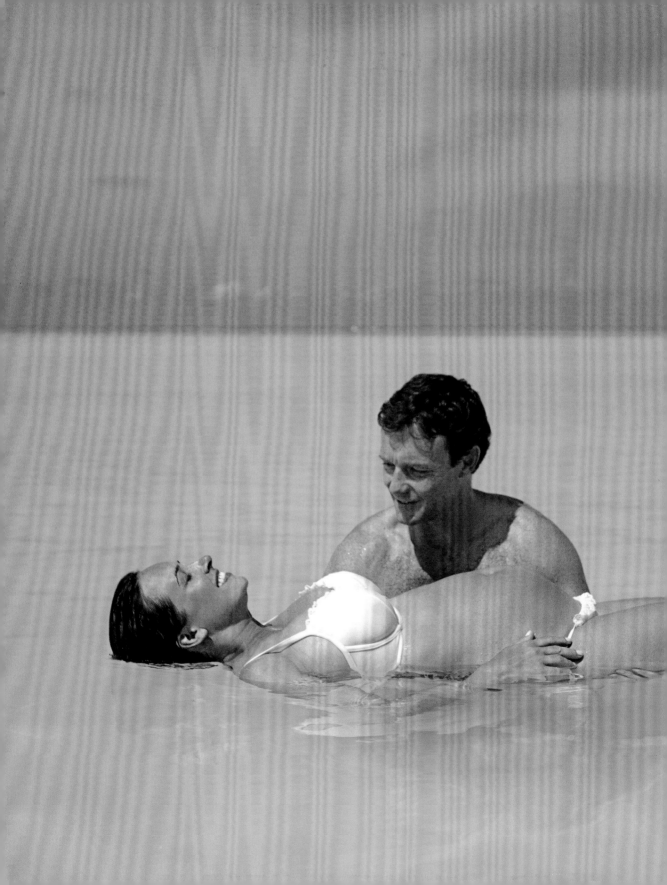

CONTENTS

{ Foreword }
by Lara Stone

Pregnancy is supposed to be the most amazing time in a woman's life. We've all heard stories of the glowing expectant mum, with the toned legs and neat bump and the instant and deep connection with her unborn baby. I'm sure those pregnancies exist, but mine certainly wasn't like that...

I was in maternity jeans at nine weeks. I was bloated all over, had limp greasy hair, no energy and I could eat (and waddle) for England. I felt terrible for feeling this way because I actually had an easy pregnancy – I had no morning sickness, no bleeding, no pain and my baby and I were perfectly healthy. Yet I didn't get that earth mother feeling I'd been hoping for.

Like a lot of women, I wanted to stay in shape during my pregnancy. But you know what? We're only human. So while we know that we need only an extra 200 calories a day towards the end of the pregnancy, if – like me – you only want to eat deep-fried food, then so be it. The most important thing during pregnancy is to grow a little person inside of you which, when you think about it, is the most amazing miracle in the world.

There is so much pressure these days to look fantastic during pregnancy and to lose the baby weight within days of leaving hospital. I have nothing against those who do, but it's not normal. Your body changes hugely during a pregnancy and it takes time to go back.

My son is now nearly five months old and my body still isn't back to how it was.

I've had lots of ups and downs regarding my body image over the past year. On every level I know I should just be happy to have a lovely healthy baby, and I do count my blessings every day. But seeing articles about me that say, 'She's brave to go outside looking like that,'

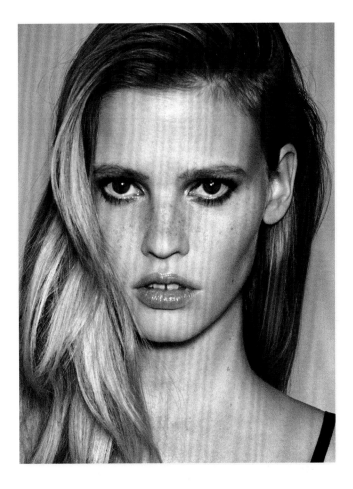

'She's struggling with her baby weight,' 'Is she pregnant again?' or 'She can kiss her career goodbye' is painful. And it sends a bad message to other women reading it, who may be feeling bad about their own baby weight.

It's been a struggle to accept the changes in my body but I've eaten Clean & Lean and tried to make time for exercise and I now feel happier, stronger and more confident. I'm still not in my pre-pregnancy jeans and I'm a few pounds heavier than I was pre-baby, but that's OK. I'm happier than ever and I love every minute of being a mum. And I no longer feel the jealous need to unfollow friends who post bikini selfies ten days after giving birth looking amazing! Because everything is just how it's supposed to be.'

INTRODUCTION

I want this book to be your best friend. I want you to feel safe and supported while you read it and I want you to take it everywhere you go so that if you need a little reminder of how amazing you are, or if you need some guidance, it's right there next to you. I want you to share it with your family and I definitely recommend that your partner reads this book as well so you can really experience this journey together.

This book isn't about losing weight, it's about teaching you to be kind to yourself and to focus on your health and the health of your beautiful, precious baby. The good news is when you do this, the weight will fall off effortlessly and you will feel strong, healthy and vibrant. We've also included guidance and tips to get you through every stage of pregnancy as well as the first 12 weeks after you've given birth.

This is the book Christiane needed when she was pregnant. It has been written to remind you that being pregnant and having a child is a wonderful, natural process, that there is nothing to be afraid of and that what is happening to you is happening to thousands of women all over the world at this very moment. Obviously I'm a man and, as such, I simply can't understand what you're going through as a woman, which is why I've brought together some of the most talented, inspiring and amazing women in the world to create this book and to provide the blueprint for a happy, safe and healthy pregnancy and beyond.

We've included stories from beautiful, brave mothers from all over the world and all walks of life. They are there for you to read when you feel lonely and will remind you of the wonderful sisterhood you belong to.

I was Christiane's birth partner and, with the help of our amazing midwife, Julie, I helped deliver our little girl Charlotte. It was the proudest and most 'alive' moment of my life. Even now, as I write this, I'm overcome with love and emotion and I have to go for a sobbing, snotty walk to get myself together. Watching my wife go through labour

My favourite pregnancy conversation: Me: 'Christiane, do you think hormones may be affecting your mood?' Christiane: 'No, James, you're just getting more annoying.'

and give birth gave me a deep sense of awe and gratitude. And as I witnessed her holding our newborn child, standing naked, fierce and beautiful, covered in blood after six hours of primal screams and heroic effort I decided two things; one, this is the strongest most wonderful person I've ever known, truly a warrior. Two, I would never, ever mess with her... ever.

I felt completely at peace as I held my hour-old little girl in my arms and for the first time in my life I knew exactly why I was alive. I felt a deep sense of duty to this little person and I was instinctively and fiercely protective of my family. I loved them both more than I could understand and my father, who had just survived lung cancer, was sitting in the next room waiting to meet the little angel he had stayed alive to see.

Life was good. And then Christiane started to lose blood. A lot of blood. A feeling of helplessness and panic filled every part of me but within seconds, Julie had dealt with the situation and saved Christiane's life. We were lucky and it was in that moment I made a commitment to help as many people come in to this world safely and with support. Our beautiful friend Teresa Palmer (Charlotte's Godmother) put us in touch with Christy Turlington and EMC (the Every Mother Counts charity). It is such a blessing to be able to help and contribute to such a wonderful cause that is very close to our hearts.

So please remember that you're not alone, that you are amazing, that you deserve a happy, healthy life and so does your baby. Thank you for giving me and Christiane the opportunity to help you and share our knowledge and the knowledge and experience of so many wonderful people that have contributed to this book. Sending you lots of love and hugs. And just know this – it's all worth it.

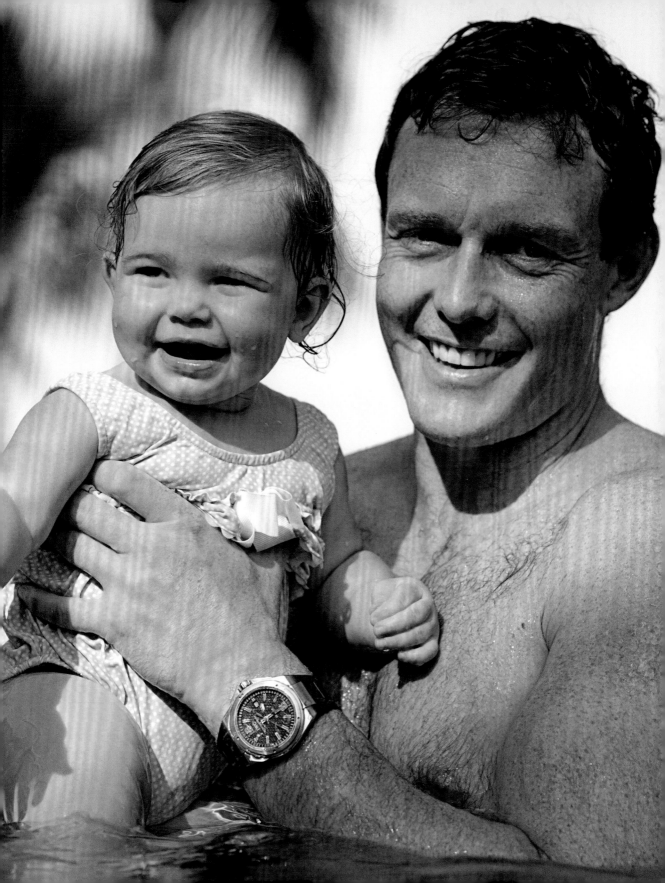

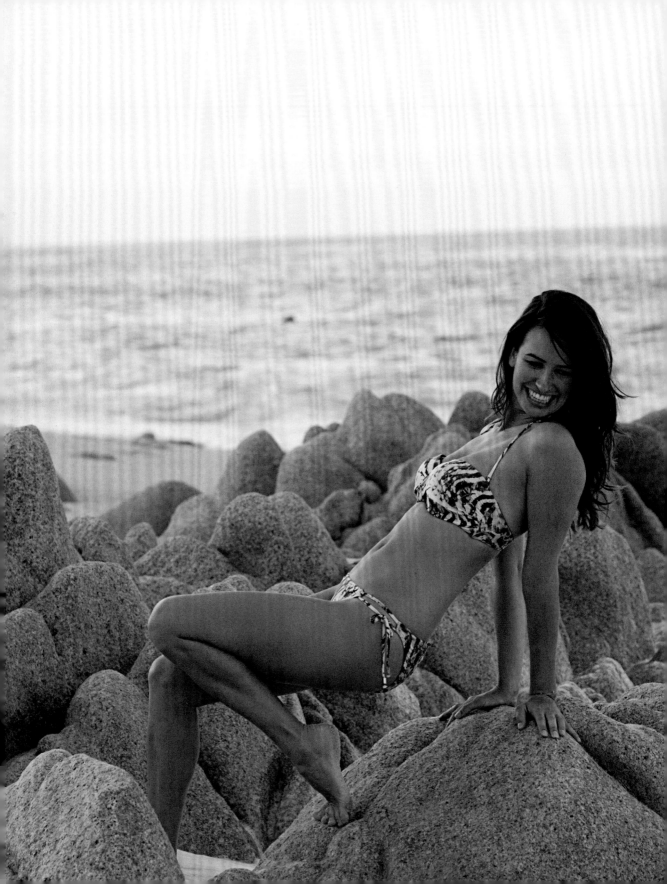

CHAPTER 1

WHAT IS CLEAN & LEAN?

CLEAN & LEAN PREGNANCY

In 2009 I wrote my first book, *The Clean & Lean Diet.* 'Clean & Lean' describes the perfect state for your body – 'clean' of fattening toxins and 'lean' as a result of a nourishing diet and regular exercise. That book became an instant bestseller and I've since written three more about the Clean & Lean way of life: one on how to get a flat tummy, another aimed at men and a recipe book. And now I bring you Clean & Lean for mums and mums-to-be.

I've spent years working with women who are either trying to get pregnant, trying to stay healthy during their pregnancies, or trying to get back in shape after having one or several babies. Those women – along with supermodel Lara Stone and the actresses Holly Valance and Teresa Palmer, whom I've had the pleasure of training with and knowing for years, and also our great friend Megan Gale – are going to share their stories of pregnancy and motherhood too. Because while it's one thing telling somebody how to stay Clean & Lean, it's another thing telling a new mum – who is sleep, time and energy deprived, and would rather be bonding with her precious new baby (or sleeping) than exercising.

Good intentions often go out the window when you're tired, craving coffee and don't have any time for yourself. This really came home to me when my wife Christiane was pregnant with and subsequently gave birth to our beautiful daughter Charlotte in 2012. I saw first-hand just how challenging it can be to eat healthily when you have morning sickness and just want to eat buttered white bread and chocolate all day. Or how difficult it can be to create a nutritious meal when you have a baby on your hip, one hand free and just five minutes to make breakfast before the next round of feeding and nappy-changing begins.

So I came up with this book – the *Clean & Lean Pregnancy Guide*. It's about self-acceptance, being kind to yourself and embracing the changes that your body is going through. It's not all about looking great – it's about feeling great. My aim is to take everything I know – from years of experience working with thousands of women all over the world, as well as from watching Christiane get her body back – and help women stay in the best possible shape and feel amazing, but in a realistic way.

So I'm not going to give you complicated healthy recipes that you don't have time to make. Neither am I going to suggest that you try to ping back into your jeans six weeks after giving birth because, frankly, it's unlikely and possibly unsafe. Instead, I'm going to give you practical advice that you can follow at your own pace, while enjoying your baby and resting.

If you eat great, you'll feel great, and that's vital when you're facing the physical and emotional challenges of pregnancy and motherhood.

This is absolutely not a diet book and I can't stress that enough. No pregnant woman or new mum should be dieting or thinking about restricting their food intake. In fact, when I use the word 'diet' in all my books, it doesn't mean what most people think: 'diet' is the way you eat, not something you do for a week to lose weight. I want you to change your diet, not 'go on' one. We should all change our eating habits so we feel great, pregnant or not. But pregnant women and new mums in particular need to focus on eating wholesome, delicious, nutritious foods that are full of goodness so that they – and their babies – stay healthy and feel amazing. Because if you eat great, you'll feel great, and that's vital when you're facing the physical and emotional challenges of pregnancy and motherhood.

So please don't think of Clean & Lean as a diet in the weight-loss sense. It's a way of eating and a way of living. Let go of guilt and don't concern yourself with 'right or wrong' or 'good and bad'. Simply focus on what works for you and embrace this experience and just celebrate how amazing you are for creating, carrying and giving birth to new life.

This book is a blueprint for a happy, healthy pregnancy and a beautiful body. It covers everything from how to increase your chances of getting pregnant, to how to eat and move right in each trimester, to getting your body back afterwards and feeling fantastic along the way. **But first, here's a quick reminder of my Clean & Lean philosophy.**

CLEAN & LEAN PHILOSOPHY

In a nutshell, your body will always struggle to be lean unless it's clean. And toxins stored in the body's fat cells will prevent that. If you're dieting, but toxic, your body might lose fat, but these toxins will have nowhere to go except back into your system. You'll feel tired, lethargic and you may have headaches, which is why most of us feel terrible soon after starting a diet. So if you're toxic, you'll always struggle to lose weight. And ironically, many diets make us more toxic with all their low-fat/high-sugar advice, so the cycle of yo-yo dieting continues.

However, if you stick to 'clean' foods, you'll look and feel great. And this is what I mean when I talk about 'clean' foods:

✳ They haven't changed much from their natural state. For example, that apple in your fruit bowl looks like it did when it was hanging on the tree. Yet crisps and bread don't look like they did in the beginning. That's because they've been processed to the point of being unrecognisable. So clean foods are those that haven't been tampered with too much.

✳ They don't have any added fake flavourings, nor are they sweetened with sugary ingredients. Their natural flavour is all that's needed to make them taste great. Succulent steak, in-season greens like asparagus, sweet berries, creamy eggs… clean foods don't need artificial flavours to make them taste good; they're delicious just as they are.

✳ They won't last for months and months. Clean foods develop mould quite quickly because they're natural and not processed with life-lengthening preservatives. A shop-bought muffin with a month-long expiry date clearly contains something that's keeping it fresh – that's most definitely not clean.

✳ They don't have a long list of ingredients, many of which you can't even pronounce, let alone recognise. Get into the habit of checking ingredients, reading labels and avoiding foods that have lengthy ingredient lists. This doesn't take long and isn't difficult – just scan the list and eat only things you know are good for you.

✳ They don't list sugar among their first three ingredients. I'm going to talk a lot about sugar in this book. We're slowly becoming more aware of just how toxic sugar is – it's fattening and makes you tired – and how it's hidden in all sorts of foods. Keep an eye out for it.

The BASICS

In order to become Clean & Lean, you'll need to familiarise yourself with just a few basic rules.

CUT BACK ON THE CRAP*

*(that's Caffeine, Refined sugar, Alcohol and Processed foods)

There are four main toxins that cause our bodies to hold on to fat.

C IS FOR CAFFEINE

This is OK in small doses. Even in pregnancy, official guidelines say you can have 200mg of caffeine or one or two cups of coffee a day. High levels of caffeine, however, can result in your baby having a low birthweight, which is associated with an increased risk of health problems later in life. Too much caffeine has also been linked to an increased miscarriage risk. So try not to exceed the 200mg limit per day, and drink plenty of still filtered water instead, because you need to stay hydrated when you're pregnant for your own health and your baby's.

Green tea is full of health-boosting antioxidants. However, it also contains caffeine, so limit yourself to three cups a day and don't drink it at all after lunch as it will disrupt your sleep, which is the last thing you need when you're pregnant or a mum. Another reason I tell clients to limit their caffeine intake is that it can put stress on the body, and when we're stressed, we release a hormone called cortisol which encourages our body to cling to fat.

New mums should also be wary of too much coffee because it can actually make them more tired (I'll talk more about this in Chapter 6). Coffee is also a diuretic – meaning it makes you urinate a lot – which can leave you feeling dehydrated and deplete your body of key

HERE'S A QUICK CAFFEINE GUIDE:

It is recommended that your daily caffeine intake does not exceed 200mg. Here's how different drinks compare:

* 1 cup of instant coffee: 100mg
* 1 cup of filter coffee: 140mg
* 1 cup of green tea: 50mg (varies between brands)
* 1 cup of tea: 75mg
* 1 can of cola: 40mg
* 1 x 50g bar of milk chocolate: 25mg

pregnancy nutrients, like calcium and iron.

It's also a good idea to reduce caffeine intake gradually when you're trying to get pregnant. Switch to decaffeinated teas and coffees and boost your energy levels in others ways: snack between meals (see p. 126 for ideas), do gentle exercise (see Chapter 2) and improve your sleep (see also Chapter 2).

R IS FOR REFINED SUGAR

In a nutshell, sugar makes you fat and tired and even though it often comes in an attractive package (cakes, biscuits, chocolate and fizzy drinks), there really is nothing to love about it. It ages us inside and out and makes us put on weight. In fact, sugar converts to bodily fat faster than fat itself because it raises insulin levels, which in turn causes excess fat to be stored. Studies show that 40 per cent of the sugar you eat is converted straight to fat, and that's if you're slim; if you're overweight, up to 60 per cent is converted to fat and stored around your stomach, waist and hips.

As I've already mentioned, sugar makes you tired and, in pregnancy, you feel tired enough already. It leaches vitamins and minerals from your body, too, making you feel hungry and weakening your immune system. A little bit of fresh, homemade cake is fine if you really fancy it, but try to avoid consuming a lot of processed sugar in drinks, low-fat yogurts and sauces on a daily basis.

A IS FOR ALCOHOL

Advice on drinking alcohol in pregnancy changes all the time, but the general consensus is that it's best to avoid it or limit it to very small amounts, such as one to two units a week. I'm not a fan of alcohol in general, let alone in pregnancy, so my take on this one is to avoid it altogether. Why take the risk?

We know that alcohol passes through the placenta and reaches your baby. When you're pregnant, your body also has to work hard to process alcohol out of your system. Excessive alcohol in pregnancy can cause miscarriage, premature birth and foetal alcohol syndrome (the effects of which can range from learning difficulties to behavioural problems to facial defects and offspring being permanently small for their age). On a lesser note, why drink something in pregnancy that's going to make you feel even more tired and crave more sugar than you already do? Your body is working hard enough during this time, creating a little person, so don't put it under even more stress.

As for new mums who are tempted to have a glass of wine every night to 'relax' – I say don't. Alcohol disrupts sleep and causes blood-sugar levels to swing, resulting in tiredness, so it's a bad way to relax. And like caffeine, alcohol puts stress on your system.

Alcohol is also full of sugar and makes you fat around the middle. I call alcohol – especially sugary wine – a 'fat bomb' that explodes all over your hips, thighs, stomach and face. I can always tell when a woman drinks too much because, no matter how slim the rest of her body is, she has 'alcohol bloat' around her face and stomach. Remember, too, that the liver is a fat-burning organ, so when it's processing alcohol, it stops burning fat. In short, alcohol leaves you squidgy, so ditch it – or at least (when you're no longer pregnant) cut right back. Find other ways to relax, like resting (when you can), warm baths, gentle exercise, reading, meditation or music.

P IS FOR PROCESSED FOODS

These go against every Clean & Lean rule there is. The less a food has been altered, the 'cleaner' it is. Clean foods include fruit, vegetables, eggs, meat (lean proteins), fish, nuts and seeds; processed foods, on the other hand, are usually made in factories, stripped of their natural goodness and pumped full of man-made preservatives and additives to make them look appetising and last longer. So stay away from tinned foods, white bread, pasta and rice, ready meals, most breakfast cereals and frozen chips and wedges. When you're a new mum it's tempting to grab quick foods, but they'll make you more tired because they don't contain enough nutrients. Instead, go for quick and healthy meals – see Chapter 8 for delicious recipes.

MEGAN GALE

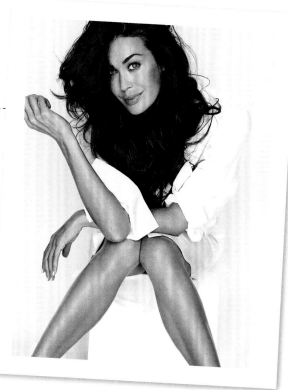

'Before I got pregnant, I had a fairly healthy body image. I've never been super-skinny or overweight – I've just tried to maintain a balance when it comes to food, diet and exercise. When Shaun and I started trying to conceive I gave up alcohol, although I've never been a big drinker. I also gave up coffee, my biggest vice. Although since then my midwife has said one to two cups of coffee a day is acceptable. However, with coffee I think it's always good to limit it if you can.

'I'm really enjoying the whole experience of being pregnant, even when I don't feel so great! I had a bit of nausea at the six-to-eight-week mark and felt exhausted. Then I got a cold, then flu, went on antibiotics and then had a chest infection which hung around until week 13. I'm now 15 weeks and feel much better, but if I've had a busy day my belly starts to feel swollen and heavy, which I think is bub's way of telling me to take it easy, so when it happens I take some time out and just rest.

'People ask whether I find it hard, as a model, to watch my body change. But I just find it mind-blowing to discover what our bodies are capable of. Like most women, I find some days it can be hard to get your head around the weight gain and expanding waistline. But I just remind myself why it's happening and how wonderful that reason is. It's also a reminder of how primal we really are. During pregnancy and motherhood, a woman's intuition is at an all-time

During pregnancy and motherhood, a woman's intuition is at an all-time high, so try to tap into that and instinctively do what feels right for you.

high, so try to tap into that and instinctively do what feels right for you.

'When it comes to losing the baby weight, women are often in a lose/lose situation. Especially women in the public eye – if they carry the baby weight for too long, they're criticised for losing their figure. If they get back to their pre-baby shape too quickly, it's implied they've been excessively dieting and exercising and are obsessed with being thin again and not thinking about their baby. They can't win. And I'm not even going to concern myself with any of that – I'm just going to concentrate on bonding with my baby.

And I can't wait!'

FAT DOESN'T MAKE YOU FAT

Don't be fat phobic! There are different types of fat: good, clean fats are the heart-friendly kind found in nuts, avocados, oily fish and oils; bad fats are found on the edge of a slice of bacon, speckled through a processed meat or in a pie crust, for example, and they should be avoided. So when I say eat more fat, I mean good fat. Good, clean fats should be eaten every day. For one thing, they help your body to absorb vitamins and minerals more efficiently, and this is incredibly important during pregnancy. For this reason, always add good fat to a salad, as it'll help your body to absorb all the goodness from the lettuce, peppers and cucumbers. Good fats also reduce sugar cravings, lift your energy levels, improve your ability to concentrate and keep you feeling full for longer. And as if all that weren't enough, they also plump up your skin and make your hair shine. In pregnancy, omega-3 fatty acids – found in oily fish – also help your baby's brain development.

WHERE ARE TOXINS FOUND?

* Sugar
* Alcohol
* Fizzy drinks
* Processed food
* Processed 'diet' food
* Excess caffeine

*top tip

While you are pregnant try to only have organic whole milk as other milks can contain growth hormones and antibiotics, which can be passed on to your baby!

WHAT ABOUT VEGETARIANS?

Clean & Lean is easy for vegetarians. Simply include lots of vegetarian proteins in your diet such as legumes, beans, lentils and chickpeas, and rather than rely too heavily on bread and pasta, choose grains such as quinoa, oats and wild rice. Also have lots of good fats from avocados, walnuts, pecans, almonds, Brazil nuts and sesame, flax and pumpkin seeds.

So that, in a nutshell, is what Clean & Lean is. It's a fairly simple way of eating and living. Just remember – if it didn't once fly, swim or walk, or wasn't pulled from the ground, from a bush or a plant, don't eat it! And you don't have to get this right 100 per cent of the time; if you aim for just 80 per cent, you'll be OK.

As I'll explain over the next eight chapters, during pregnancy, more than ever, you need to listen to your body. But remember, if you're pregnant, everything you eat, drink and do, your baby is experiencing too. I'm not saying that to make you feel guilty – I'm saying it so you'll treat your own body and health during pregnancy in the same way as you'll treat your baby's once they are born. You want only the best for them, so they feel good and grow up healthy, and you need to treat yourself just as kindly. It's the same for new mums – I've seen so many who feed their baby puréed organic vegetables, while they have coffee and chocolate themselves.

You deserve to be looked after too and that's what this book is all about. Good luck!

CLEAN & LEAN FOODS

CLEAN & LEAN PROTEINS

Great sources of protein:
* Chicken
* Turkey
* Lamb
* Beef
* Duck
* All fish (but remember: just two servings of oily fish a week in pregnancy and no shark, marlin or swordfish)

And for vegetarians:
* Eggs
* Beans
* Lentils
* Nuts
* Seeds
* Yogurt
* Cheese

*top tip

Freeze your fruit! Wash and cover bite-sized pieces of fruit – such as whole grapes and blueberries, halved strawberries and chunks of pineapple – and place in the freezer. When you feel like something sweet or fancy ice-cream or a lolly, try some frozen fruit instead to satisfy your sweet craving.

CLEAN & LEAN FLAVOURS

The more fresh flavours you put into your food, the better it will taste and the easier it will be to avoid all those nasty fake flavours in the form of processed sugar and additives.

Here are some ideas:
* Avocado oil
* Basil-infused oil
* Coconut oil
* First-press extra virgin olive oil (the best that you can buy)
* Flaxseed oil
* Sesame oil
* Walnut oil
* Garlic-infused olive oil
* White wine vinegar
* Delouis Fils mayonnaise (keep refrigerated)
* Dijon mustard
* Tamari (gluten- and sugar- and salt-free)
* Lemons
* Limes
* Garlic
* Coriander
* Dill
* Oregano
* Parsley
* Thyme
* Chilli
* Cinnamon
* Cayenne pepper
* Turmeric

And here are some of my own personal favourite flavours that deserve a special mention:

* Cinnamon can reduce blood-sugar levels and, therefore, sugar cravings and bad cholesterol. It's also an anti-inflammatory, so it can help with aches and pains. Sprinkle ground cinnamon on your coffee or porridge.
* Garlic helps with so many things. It's antiviral, so it wards off colds and boosts your immune system, plus it's an antioxidant and lowers bad cholesterol.
* Ginger is a great antioxidant. It's also been shown to boost the immune system, help blood circulation and aid digestion. Slice some of the root into hot water with a squeeze of lemon to make a refreshing drink.
* Parsley helps the kidneys flush out toxins, plus it freshens your breath. It's also good for keeping blood-sugar levels steady.
* Rosemary is great for your brain and is used by aromatherapists the world over to improve mood.

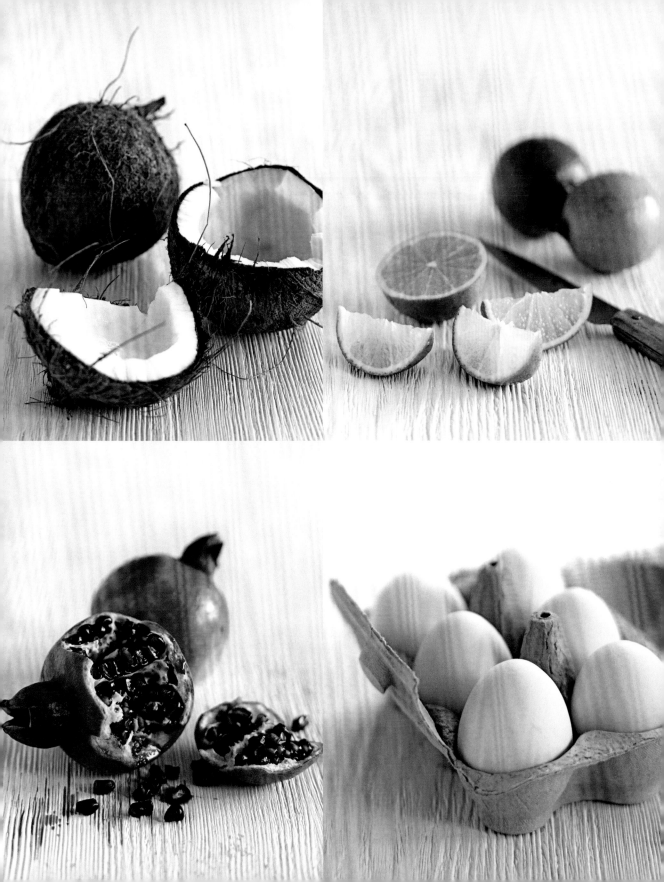

CLEAN & LEAN VEGETABLES

Vegetables that are organic and in season contain twice as many vitamins as those that are not. Try local farmers' markets, and if you can't afford to buy organic, always try to buy in-season. Out-of-season vegetables have often been flown for miles, so are sprayed with life-lengthening preservatives and may contain fewer nutrients.

The following vegetables are good choices:

* Asparagus
* Avocado
* Broccoli
* Brussels sprouts
* Butternut squash
* Carrots
* Cauliflower
* Courgette
* Cucumber
* Green beans
* Kale
* Mangetout
* Peppers
* Rocket
* Spinach
* Sweet potato
* Watercress

CLEAN & LEAN NUTS & SEEDS

Eat raw nuts whenever possible – the roasting process can cause nuts to go rancid, which increases free-radical damage in your body. Try the following:

Nuts
* Almonds
* Brazil nuts
* Cashews
* Chestnuts
* Macadamia nuts
* Peanuts
* Pecans
* Pistachios
* Walnuts

Seeds
* Chia
* Flax
* Linseed
* Pumpkin
* Sesame
* Sunflower

*top tip

Make a big portion of your favourite meal, divide it up into containers and keep some in the fridge and some in the freezer – perfect for those days (and especially evenings) when you're too tired to cook, but fancy something filling and nutritious.

TRY THIS DIP

Mash up and mix half an avocado, a dollop of full-fat Greek yogurt, some crushed garlic, chopped fresh coriander, chopped jalapeño chilli, lime juice, ground cumin, salt and pepper. Eat on its own or with oatcakes or rye bread.

TERESA PALMER

'Ever since I was a little girl all I've longed for is to become a mother. I had an old-fashioned pram and I filled it with dolls and lugged it around everywhere. Now I'm 27 and expecting my first child, a son, with my husband Mark.

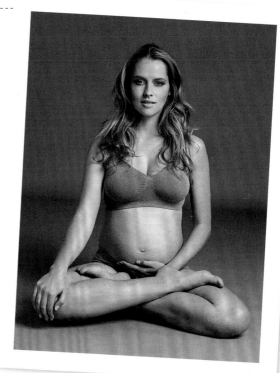

'It took us seven months to get pregnant, which doesn't sound like a long time. But it felt like an eternity, as anybody who has tried, or is trying, to get pregnant will know. I'd spent my whole adult life trying not to get pregnant but then, when I wanted to, it wasn't that easy. I was disappointed with my body and felt a lot of despair.

'Once I was pregnant the self-judgement didn't stop. I placed huge expectations on myself and felt guilty if I ate something "bad." Before I got pregnant I told myself I'd be the healthiest pregnant woman ever – nothing processed and nothing fried would pass my lips. But I was shocked to discover that's exactly what I craved – I just wanted chips and sweets!

'Pregnancy wasn't at all how I'd expected it to be. But that's the problem right there – placing an expectation on how things "should" be. Once I freed myself from expectation, I began to enjoy my pregnancy and the changes it bought. I marvelled at the aches and pains I experienced and my protruding belly. Once I sat back and allowed the experience of pregnancy to come to me – without trying to control it – I felt more rooted. It's the art of surrendering – observing your body and trusting it to tell you what it needs.

'I didn't exercise at all during the first trimester – I was too exhausted and chose sleep instead because I listened to my body. After 12 weeks, I started Pilates and yoga. It was beautiful to regain some strength. I freed myself from guilt about what I ate too, and had what I wanted but in a mindful

Once I allowed the experience of pregnancy to come to me, I felt more rooted. It's the art of observing your body and trusting it to tell you what it needs.

way. I had a green juice every day and a plant-based prenatal vitamin supplement, so if I made a few unhealthy diet choices they balanced things out.

'The day we saw our little man doing somersaults on the ultrasound scan was the most special feeling I've ever had. We had created this little being! And those tiny toes we were watching wriggling on the screen were the very same toes we would be kissing in a few months' time. It bought home to me just how miraculous a journey pregnancy is. It's so special, so surreal, and yet so natural.

'Lastly, I believe all women have the right to have birthing options and be able to have their best birth possible. Whichever path you choose – medicated, non-medicated, in a hospital environment or at home – you know how best to birth your own baby.'

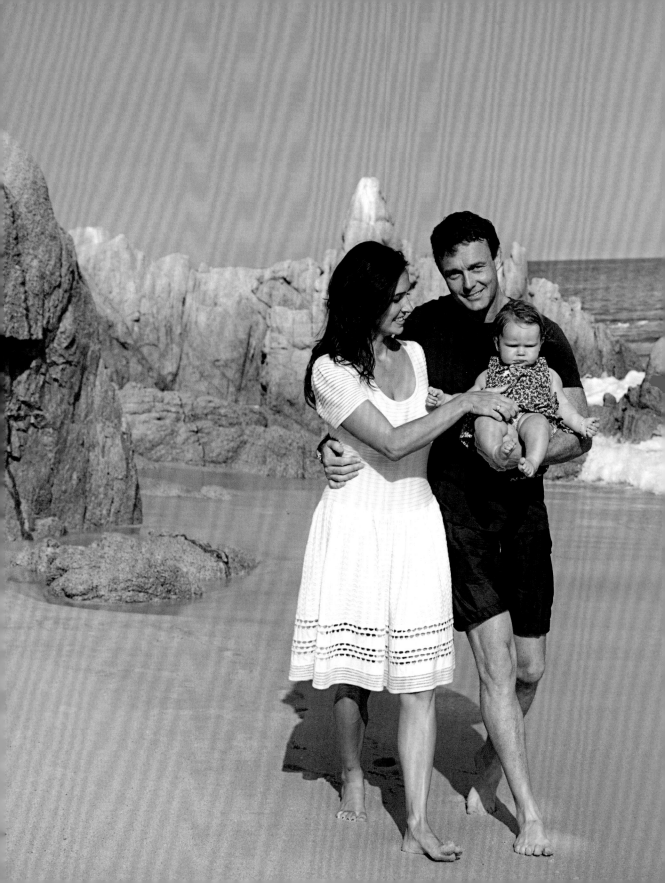

CHAPTER 2

HOW TO BOOST, PROTECT & EXTEND YOUR FERTILITY

I couldn't write a book about pregnancy without addressing the fact that getting pregnant in the first place isn't easy for everybody. Nothing brought this home to me more than when my wife Christiane and I struggled to conceive our daughter Charlotte. We were both young and healthy, so took our fertility for granted, never imagining it could take so long.

There is still so much to discover about why some people become pregnant easily and others don't. But what we do know is that there are several steps you can take to help you along the way. As Christiane and I prove, being healthy isn't a guarantee of fertility, but countless studies do link a healthy lifestyle to increased fertility, so making the right changes to your life will improve your chances. And taking control of your fertility is important, because when you're trying and failing to conceive you often feel powerless.

So this chapter, based on a combination of my work with clients who were trying to get pregnant, our own experience and the advice of some fantastic experts we met during that time, is my guide to increasing, protecting and extending your fertility.

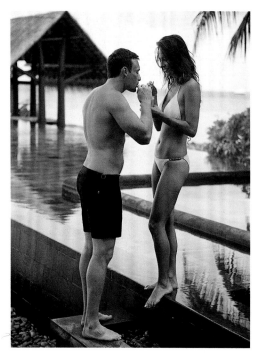

INFERTILITY EXPLAINED

Jane is a world-renowned fertility specialist and Clinical Director of the Acupuncture IVF Support Clinic (www.acupunctureivf.com.au). She helps couples going through IVF to conceive with the help of Chinese herbs and acupuncture and she's amazing – she supported Christiane and me through a very difficult time. There are some experts who just stand out and Jane is one of them. We can't thank her enough.

'I see a lot of unexplained infertility, like James and Christiane's, in my clinic. But what might be unexplained in orthodox medical terms may well have an explanation in Chinese medicine, which looks at more subtle and whole body factors. Infertility is "unexplained" if a couple has not conceived in a year of trying, and neither partner has been diagnosed with a condition which would affect their fertility. This includes, for women, endometriosis, polycystic ovarian disease, age (older than 38 years), tubal blockage or autoimmune conditions. For men infertility is diagnosed by certain parameters measured in a semen analysis which relate to the number of sperm, their shape, how well they swim and the integrity of their DNA.

'When couples struggle to conceive – for whatever reason – they often feel incredibly frustrated. Sometimes having a label which leads to a definitive treatment is an easier diagnosis to cope with. However, treatments for many of the conditions that lead to infertility do not have simple and straightforward treatments with guaranteed outcomes.

'Whether or not couples can help themselves depends on the cause of their infertility, but generally there is much couples can do to improve their fertility. Let's start with men, because it is often easier to improve sperm than it is eggs. Lifestyle factors make a big difference to the health of sperm, and the good news is that most of it is under your control. Heavy alcohol consumption has a deleterious effect on sperm count and function, but moderate drinking seems to do no harm. All relevant studies have shown the negative effects of tobacco or marijuana on sperm. If you're having difficulty giving up either of these, seek help immediately if you're trying to conceive. As for coffee, a little bit is fine for most men, but more than three cups a day has been shown to damage sperm DNA. Being overweight is associated with decreased testosterone and increased oestrogen, neither of which is good news for your sperm count or quality. Now is a good time to start a weight-loss programme. Acupuncture can help control your appetite and accelerate weight loss.

'Frequent sex improves the quality of sperm, while a few days' abstinence increases the quantity of sperm. So when the woman is ovulating, daily sex around this time is recommended. If not, have sex every second day from when her period finishes and continue for ten days (or more if she has a long cycle). We also know that men exposed to chemicals or fumes at their work place have lower sperm counts, so try your best to limit exposure. We know that electromagnetic radiation from mobile phones and laptops is associated with hormone changes and that long hours of use are associated with reduced fertility. Do not keep your mobile phone in the side pocket of your trousers and try to limit its use.

'Lastly, a number of clinical studies have shown the beneficial effects of acupuncture and Chinese herbs in improving sperm quality and fertility. More than ten separate trials in a number of different countries have all shown a significant improvement in sperm morphology and motility after a course of acupuncture.

'For women, the underlying cause (if there is one) needs to be addressed. Endometriosis is usually treated with surgery, and polycystic ovarian disease is often treated with drugs that reduce insulin levels (diabetes drugs) and drugs to induce ovulation if necessary. We don't yet have effective drug treatments for autoimmune conditions, except steroids which may be used in some situations. For age-related infertility, there is no drug treatment, although DHEA as a supplement might improve egg quality. Chinese medicine offers very good proven treatments for endometriosis and polycystic ovarian disease.

Generally there is much couples can do to improve their fertility.

'In my clinic we see couples with infertility and assess them from a Chinese medicine point of view. This means taking a thorough case history and looking at what investigations have been done already. All aspects of the body and mind are taken into account with a focus on the reproductive system, of course. Sometimes it is clear that Chinese medicine will not help improve fertility (for example, if the fallopian tubes are blocked) and we will refer the couple to an IVF clinic if they wish to take that route.

'For most conditions related to infertility, including those that don't have a Western medicine label, a Chinese medicine programme can be formulated and we can expect good results. We use Chinese herbs, which are taken twice daily as a tea (a rather strong-tasting tea, but most people get used to it quickly). Acupuncture is done weekly or fortnightly, in the case of women for 3–6 months. For men we treat once or twice a week, for 1–3 months, and then retest the sperm. Sometimes we work together with the IVF clinic to prepare a couple who have had previous IVF failures, in the hope that their chances are better with subsequent cycles.

'We probably see as much secondary infertility as we do primary infertility. These couples are particularly frustrated because they know they have achieved pregnancy at least once before. Often the cause is unexplained from a Western medicine point of view, but Chinese medicine will usually find a cause that may be related to factors that have arisen since the first child or previous children – sometimes this is depletion of internal resources or stress which can upset the hormone balance. Sometimes it is related to age. Improving lifestyle factors like stress, sleep patterns and digestion often helps with this type of infertility.

'I'm so glad I could help James and Christiane, who will share with you my advice – and plenty more from other experts and themselves – in this book. Good luck.'
BY JANE LYTTLETON BSc (Hons) NZ, MPhil Lond, Dip TCM Aus, Cert Ac, Cert Herbal Medicine, China

FERTILITY AND STRESS

For years studies have been showing that stress is linked to fertility – which can lead to a vicious cycle of feeling stressed that you're not getting pregnant, then worrying that stress is making the problem worse. People will say things like, 'Don't worry about it and it will just happen.' They'll then go on to tell you about their friend who went on holiday or who decided to adopt a baby and who then fell pregnant straight away because they had 'stopped worrying about it'.

Although well meaning, this sort of advice can be very frustrating, and yet the truth is that stress and fertility are inextricably linked, and that's why I've included it here. A few simple lifestyle changes can make a huge difference and improving your diet and regularly getting more sleep is the perfect place to start.

FOODS THAT REDUCE STRESS

✳ **Berries** are full of vitamin C, which allows the body to cope better with stress. They're also full of fibre, which helps to regulate blood-sugar levels (these can fluctuate when we're stressed).

✳ **Green vegetables** – dark green vegetables help to replenish our bodies with vitamins in times of stress.

✳ **Turkey** contains an amino acid called L-tryptophan, which releases serotonin (a calming, feel-good hormone) into the body. Eating turkey has a soothing effect on the body and can even help you sleep better.

✳ **Sweet potatoes** will satisfy a carb craving (common during stressful times, because blood-sugar level swings cause us to crave sugar fixes), and also contain more fibre and vitamins than ordinary potatoes.

✳ **Avocados** – all the good fat and potassium they contain can lower your blood pressure (which rises during times of stress).

✳ **Nuts** help to boost an immune system weakened by stress, plus they're full of B vitamins which help to lower stress levels.

FOODS THAT INCREASE STRESS

✳ **Coffee** – too much caffeine stresses out your system by constantly flooding your body with the fat-storing hormone cortisol. Stick to one or two cups of organic coffee a day.

✳ **Alcohol** stimulates the adrenal glands – two tiny glands that sit just above our kidneys and pump out the stress hormone adrenaline. Studies have also shown that alcohol reduces fertility in both sexes, so if you're trying to get pregnant, cut right back or, ideally, stop drinking altogether.

✳ **Sweets and sugary snacks** give you a quick burst of energy, but then they cause your blood-sugar levels to crash, leaving you feeling sluggish, stressed and lacking concentration.

✳ **Processed foods** are full of so much junk that they deplete the levels of vitamins and minerals in your body, leaving you more prone to stress.

✳ **Junk food** – studies show that foods that are high in bad fats (burgers, chips, kebabs, etc.) lower your concentration levels and increase your stress levels.

✳ **Salty foods** increase your blood pressure, which makes you more prone to stress. The worst offenders are processed meats like ham, bacon, and others that are full of salt.

SLEEP YOURSELF LESS STRESSED

Sleep (or a lack of it) and stress often go hand in hand. When we're stressed, we find it more difficult to sleep, and when we're tired, we feel more stressed – it's enough to make you need a nap!

I can't stress enough just how important it is to have sufficient sleep – especially if you're trying to get pregnant. Good restorative sleep is as crucial to brain function and health as are oxygen and water. However, many of us think we can get away with skimping on sleep as we pack more and more into our busy lives. Technology doesn't help matters and neither does the current trend for associating being busy with being important.

Many of us these days are working longer hours than ever and travelling more. And while all these things can enrich our lives to some extent, they can also take their toll on our health. One study from the University of Chicago has found that not sleeping enough can mimic ageing – put simply, your body ages prematurely if you don't get enough shut-eye.

So – want to know how can you sleep better? Read on.

SLEEP SMARTER...

Turn off your technology
Too many of us are ruining our sleep with technology – and I for one am guilty of this. It's easy to waste a whole evening browsing mindlessly on our iPads, phones or laptops when we could be exercising, seeing friends, having a conversation with our partner or relaxing in a nice bath. Technology was designed to save us time, but it robs us of time and this can leave us feeling stressed. It can also delay bedtime. Plus, the flickering light from screens stimulates our brains in a way that makes falling asleep afterwards more difficult.

Limit the time you spend using technology in the evenings and do something more relaxing instead. If you don't browse on your phone for an hour before bed, your sleep will automatically become deeper and leave you feeling more refreshed in the morning.

Avoid caffeine
This is so obvious I can't believe I'm saying it, but so many of us forget about the sleep-robbing effects of caffeine.

*top tip
Too many of us take our technology to bed. Keep phones, and iPads and laptops out of the bedroom!*

Never, ever be tempted by a 4pm latte. No matter how immune you think you are to the effects of caffeine, it will disrupt your sleep. It interferes with the way the body processes the enzyme adenosine that causes us to feel drowsy and fall asleep and so results in wakefulness. Lack of sleep in turn causes you to feel more stressed the next day and, ironically, more likely to rely on caffeine – and so the cycle continues. Remember, it's also found in regular tea, green tea, soft drinks, chocolate and certain medications (see p. 14).

Add a few drops of lavender oil to your evening bath
You'll fall asleep more easily. There's a reason why sleep experts tell mums to bathe their babies before bed to help them sleep better – soaking in warm water helps us to fall into a deeper sleep, according to several studies.

Stick to a routine
Try to go to bed and wake up at approximately the same time every day, even at weekends. Our sleep–wake cycle is regulated by our circadian clock – a type of internal alarm clock that reminds the brain when to release sleep and wake hormones and when not to. Keeping consistent sleep time strengthens this clock, and you'll sleep more soundly as a result.

Don't argue, worry, eat, drink alcohol or smoke...
You shouldn't be doing either of the latter anyway, if you're trying to conceive, but try not to do any of these too close to bedtime.

Keep your bedroom for sleep and sex
Sex, by the way, promotes better sleep! Orgasm releases the hormone prolactin, which leads to feelings of relaxation and sleepiness and results in a good night's sleep. Furthermore, dopamine and oxytocin are also released and these create a feeling of wellbeing, which also leads to a restful sleep.

PRE-PREGNANCY EXERCISES TO BOOST FERTILITY

There are specific muscles and movements that you are going to need in order to stay healthy, pain-free and fully functional throughout your pregnancy. This programme is designed to give you a beautiful, strong foundation for a happy, healthy pregnancy.

Perform each exercise once; the whole routine should take you only about ten minutes, and I would like you to do it every day, if possible. The message here – as it is throughout the whole of this book – is to be kind to yourself. Don't overdo exercise, especially if you're trying to get pregnant. Over-exercising can have as much of an impact on fertility as being unfit or overweight. Being underweight and not having enough body fat can affect your menstrual cycle and your ability to become pregnant.

As you do the exercises in this chapter, repeat this little mantra as it will give you something positive to focus on, and I promise it will make you feel better:

'I'm in perfect health, I'm ready for my healthy, beautiful baby, I deserve a happy, healthy life.'

If you'd rather not use the mantra, and you think I'm a weirdo, that's fine! Just be sure to do the exercises, because they're brilliant.

Important note: Seek advice from your GP or health professional if you are in any doubt about exercising while trying to conceive.

EXERCISE	REPS	SETS	REST
Tummy vacuum	8–10	1	30 secs
Superman	10–15/side	1	30 secs
Plank	15–30-sec hold	1	30 secs
Push-up from the knees	5	1	30 secs
Y	10–15	1	60 secs

HOW TO PERFORM THE EXERCISES

Perform the following exercises at the beginning of every workout to ensure your lower back, core (see p. 31) and shoulders are activated and engaged and ready for the workout. Perform each exercise in turn, doing the stated number of repetitions and taking the stated amount of rest between each exercise. Once the final exercise is completed, move on to the circuit programme on p. 34.

Tummy vacuum

Start position: Support yourself on your hands and knees with hands under shoulders, arms straight and knees under hips. Ensure your arms and thighs remain at right angles to the floor, keep your back straight and your head aligned with your upper back.

The movement: Relax your stomach, letting it sag towards the floor while maintaining a flat back. Then squeeze your tummy muscles and pull your belly button towards the ceiling, still maintaining a flat back and hold for 5 seconds. Repeat 8–10 times.

*top tip

As you draw your belly button towards your spine, squeeze your pelvic floor muscles (that stop the flow of urine) as this helps prepare for an easier birth and recovery.

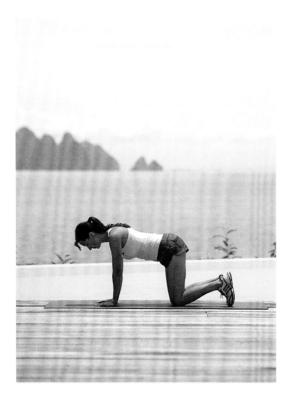

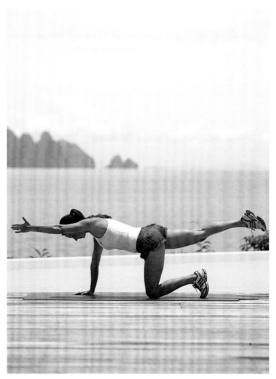

Superman

Start position: Support yourself on your hands and knees with hands under shoulders and knees under hips and with your toes firmly pointed into the floor. Ensure your spine and neck are in a straight line by keeping your gaze to the floor, just in front of your fingertips.

The movement: Extend your left arm out in front of you beyond your head, thumb up, while extending your right leg backward – imagine you are being pulled from either end. Return to the start position and repeat 10–15 times on each side.

*top tip

This exercise will activate and strengthen your hamstrings, glutes and lower-back muscles, as well as improve your overall body balance.

*top tip

To set the core, pull your belly button in towards the spine so your stomach muscles are engaged.

Plank

Start position: Lie face down on the floor with forearms and elbows touching the floor, hips and legs on the ground.

The movement: Keeping your head aligned with your upper back, raise your hips and set the core. Imagine a straight line from your head to your ankles. Hold for 15–30 seconds, then return to the start position.

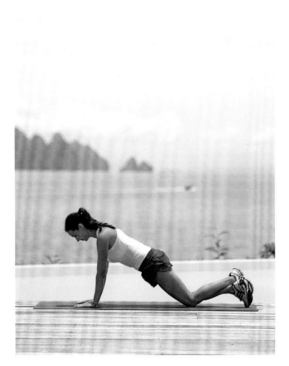

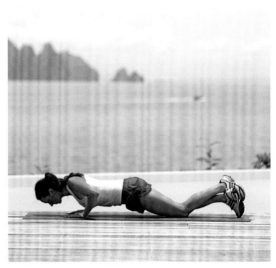

Push-up from the knees

Start position: Place your knees on the ground. Set your hands shoulder-width apart and in line with your nipples, not your shoulders. Keep your ears, shoulders and hips in alignment and your feet crossed behind you, toes down and pushing into the floor for stability. Set the core by pulling your belly button in towards the spine.

The movement: Keeping your body straight, lower yourself so your nose almost touches the ground, then lift back up to the start position. Remember to ensure that your spine and neck are in a straight line by keeping your gaze to the floor, just in front of your fingertips. Keep your belly button drawn in, then breathe out as you push up to the start position, and breathe in as you lower down. Repeat 5 times.

*top tip

Keep your belly button drawn in to help improve the connection between your brain and your tummy muscles.

If you find this too difficult, start in the same position as above but with your torso elevated with your hands on a chair or sofa. The higher up your arms are, or the less horizontal the body is, the easier the push-up will be.

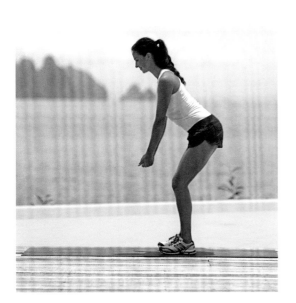
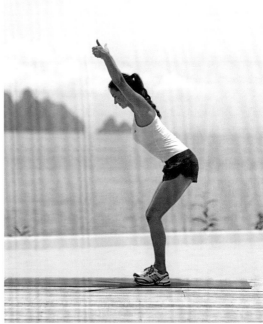

Y

Start position: With your feet hip-width apart, bend your knees and stick your bottom out, so your upper body leans forward 45 degrees. Hold your hands directly below your chest with fists clenched and thumbs up, keeping your head and back in a straight line, your shoulders back and down, and your core tight.

The movement: Raise both hands to create a 'Y' shape above your head with your arms by your ears, then return to the starting point. Repeat 10–15 times.

*top tip

Perform this exercise slowly and with control to ensure your body stays relaxed. The less the body is stressed, the easier it can be to become pregnant.

CIRCUIT TRAINING

At Bodyism, we love to get our clients to perform circuits like the one below. This type of circuit is a great way to work lots of muscles and improve your posture, as well as get a great cardiovascular workout without spending time on a bike or treadmill.

The circuit below is designed to strengthen in particular those muscles you're going to need to be robust during the early stages of your pregnancy, as well as post-pregnancy once your beautiful baby is here – your lower back, hamstrings, shoulders, back and core/tummy muscles. All of these muscle groups need to be strong to help with the added weight gained during pregnancy, as well as to help create a stable, strong body that can handle the birth process. Do each exercise, one after the other, performing the stated number of repetitions and taking the stated amount of rest between each exercise. Once the final exercise is completed, rest for 90 seconds before performing the stated number of sets.

EXERCISE	REPS	SETS	REST
Plié squat	12–15	2–3	30 secs
L to shoulder press	10–12	2–3	30 secs
Flamingo	10–12/ side	2–3	30 secs
Bent-over row (holding ball)	10–12	2–3	30 secs
Side plank	15–30-sec hold/side	2–3	60 secs

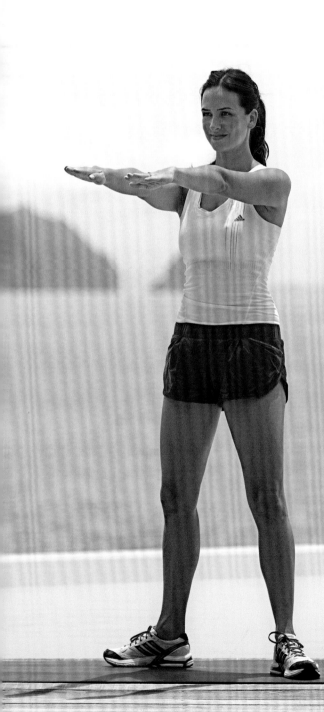

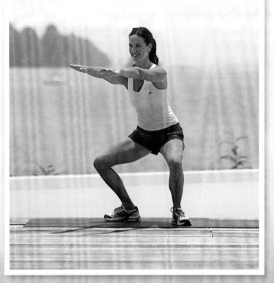

Plié squat

Start position: Stand with your arms straight out in front at shoulder height, feet shoulder-width apart and toes pointed out at 45 degrees. Keep your core engaged by pulling your belly button in towards your spine.

The movement: Keeping your arms straight, initiate the movement by pushing the hips back and bending the knees so you squat back and down until your thighs are parallel to the floor.

Return to the standing position by pushing through the hips and the heels while keeping your torso upright. Repeat 12–15 times.

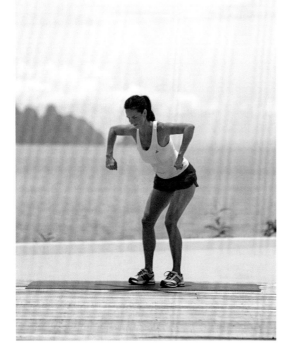

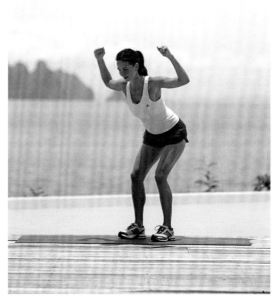

L to shoulder press

Start position: Take a comfortable stance with your feet hip-width apart. Bend your knees and stick your bottom out so your upper body hinges forward from the hips. Keep your head and back in a straight line, shoulders back and down, arms by your sides, palms facing backward. Engage your core by pulling your belly button in towards your spine.

The movement: With your core engaged, bring your arms upward, leading with your elbows until they reach shoulder height. Rotate your forearms upward until the backs of your hands face the ceiling, making an 'L' shape with your arms, then straighten your arms upward to perform a shoulder-press movement. Reverse this pattern back to the starting position and repeat 10–12 times.

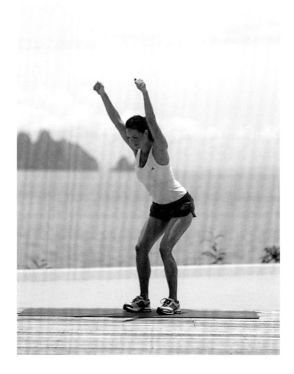

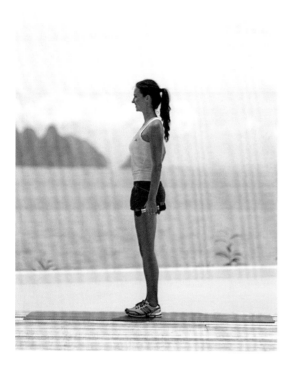

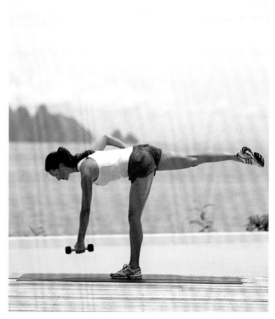

Flamingo

Start position: Stand with your feet together, right hand on your waist and the left holding a light weight by your side. Keep your core engaged by pulling your belly button in towards your spine.

The movement: Hinge over at your waist by pushing your right leg back behind you. Be sure to keep your standing leg slightly bent, while your back and neck remain in a perfect line. Return to the start position and repeat 10–12 times on each side.

*top tip

This exercise is great for strengthening your hamstrings. Perform it slowly and with control to create stability in the lower body.

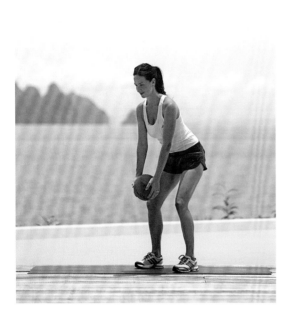
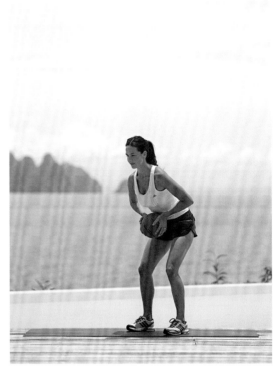

Bent-over row
(holding ball)

Start position: Stand with feet shoulder-width apart and, holding either a ball or dumbbell, hinge over at the waist. Ensure your neck and spine are in a straight line by fixing your gaze slightly down and in front of you and engage your core by pulling your belly button in towards the spine.

The movement: Slide your shoulder blades back and pull your elbows toward the sky, raising the ball or dumbbell up to your belly button. Lower the ball/dumbbell back down to the start position and repeat 10–12 times.

*top tip

This exercise targets the postural muscles in the back. Good postural alignment not only strengthens the skeletal system but also supports the body's vital organs, including the reproductive organs.

*top tip

Strong and stable core muscles can help prevent back problems during pregnancy and help towards an easier labour and quicker postpartum recovery.

Side plank

Start position: Lie on your side with your feet stacked on top of each other, your right forearm on the ground, your right elbow under your right shoulder and your left hand resting on your waist. Engage your core by pulling your belly button in towards the spine.

The movement: Keeping your elbow under your shoulder and your legs straight, lift your hips into the air so that there is a straight line from the top of your head to your heel. Keep your core engaged and hold for 15–30 seconds, then repeat on the opposite side.

SALLY OBERMEDER

'For me, being pregnant was the most amazing experience I have ever had! To know that a precious being was growing inside me with my help just made me feel so lucky and it had extra special meaning as it had taken me so long to decide when the exact right time was to have a baby and then to get pregnant. Naively, I thought that as soon as I had decided to have a baby, that it would happen straightaway. For the other big hurdles of my life – a career change and major weight loss – there was a direct correlation between effort and result, so I thought baby-making would be the same. However, after years of trying and struggling and never producing a baby, I realised that this was one of those life events that plays by a different set of rules. In the end I found success with IVF, and very fortunately after just one cycle.

'I was a little apprehensive about what my pregnancy would be like. I don't know if I was insanely lucky or just stuck floating on cloud nine, but I had no bad experiences at all – well, my boobs got huge, but I guess that's not something to complain about! No morning sickness, no weird cravings for gherkins dipped in peanut butter or hot dog hankerings at 2am. I wanted to be as healthy as I could be for myself and my much-longed-for baby. I kept up my fitness routine, adapting it to my ever-growing belly; I started Pilates classes and I truly have never felt healthier, happier or more content. I know everyone says this about their babies but she was my little miracle and already she had my spirit – even though she needed a little nudge through IVF to get here, she was a fighter and stubborn and she was going to get here one way or another.

'At the very end of my pregnancy and ironically when I was feeling my best, I was hit with the very hardest blow I have ever had. The day before Annabelle was born, I was diagnosed with stage 3 breast cancer. The cancer was both rare and

> *She was my little miracle and already she had my spirit – she was a fighter and stubborn and she was going to get here one way or another.*

aggressive and the outlook was not at all good. I knew then and there that I had no choice but to fight like a bloody warrior and make it through for my baby. We had gone through so much to get here and I couldn't let our relationship end before it had even begun.

'Chemo was tough, so tough that there were days when I really did just want to give up – to this day I don't really know exactly what it did to my husband Marcus, who was of course so worried about losing me, and yet he was always there as my rock and helping me through some of the most harrowing moments.

'And then there was Annabelle. I had so much I wanted to share with my daughter and there was no way I was going to let her grow up without a mother. Sometimes I still grieve for my first year of motherhood – it wasn't at all how I thought it would be. No playgroups or play dates with other mothers, just chemo and scans, tests and radiation, surgery and more surgery. I felt guilty that I wasn't being a "proper" mum to Annabelle but I would remind myself that I was fighting this fight with every ounce of the limited physical strength that I had, just to ensure that I would live to see her first steps, first words, her first day at school and all the firsts that every parent longs to witness.

'I am incredibly blessed to still be here today and am the happiest I've ever been. I know it's an overused phrase, but I've learnt to savour every moment, to be "in the moment". I close my eyes and take pictures with my memory and soak up every detail. I'm proud to say I have a happy, healthy 2-year-old monkey, a loving husband and amazing family and friends. I may have scars all over my body as a result of the many surgeries, but I'm proud of them and every time I look at Annabelle I think how far we've come together.'

YOGA FOR FERTILITY

Yoga has completely changed my and Christiane's life. It is difficult to express how grateful we are to the yoga experts Wenche Beard, Una Laffan and Danai Kougiouli who gave us love and support while we were trying to get pregnant and every moment since then, and who have contributed incredible routines for this book.

Una is an amazing lady. She has studied Ashtanga Vinyasa Yoga and other forms of movement and dance therapies in Mexico, the US and India and I'm so happy she is able to share her wisdom here:

'In the pre-conception stage we need to be gentle with ourselves and our bodies. Enjoy a yoga practice that nourishes and soothes your system and allows you to find space where you can slow down and ground yourself. The following sequence emphasises breath, softness and openness. It focuses on the hips and pelvis to improve the flow of energy through these parts of your body. The connection between your breath and movement will calm the mind and help you feel in touch, in tune and in love with your body. The routine is designed as a fluid progression so perform each pose and then move on to the next.'

BY UNA LAFFAN

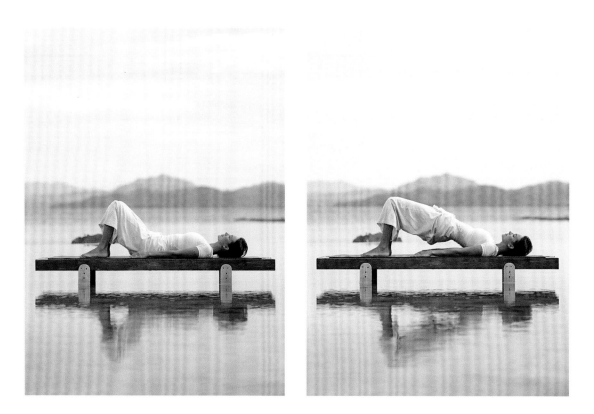

Setu Bandhasana (Supported bridge pose)

Lie on your back, knees raised, with feet hip-width apart, toes and thighs parallel, heels close to your sitting bones. Take a moment to find your breath and feel your breath soften your stomach, chest, throat and face.

As you exhale, press your feet into the earth and let your hips lift up, lengthening your tailbone towards the knees and keeping your thighs and inner feet parallel.

Without squeezing the buttocks, allow the strength of your legs and feet to support your hips and keep the breath soft into the belly. Relax your internal organs. Enjoy the opening and softening of your belly and chest area as you feel the strength and support of your legs, back and shoulders. Breathe a few rounds of breath as you connect your feet into the earth, then come down for 2 breaths. Repeat 3–4 times.

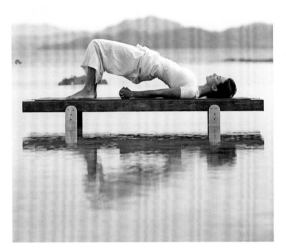
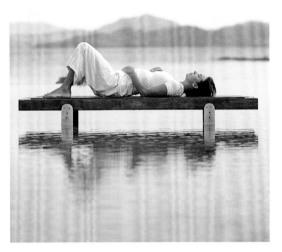

A deeper variation: When your hips are raised, interlace your hands underneath your back on the floor. Be gentle and breathe here for at least 5 breaths, as your front body softens into the support of your lower and back body. Repeat 3–4 times.

To finish, lower your hips slowly to the ground, relaxing your spine down. Take a moment to rest with one palm on your lower belly and the other on your heart. Feel the breath under your palms as you soften your jaw, heart and belly. Rest and delight in your breath until you feel your body is ready to move on.

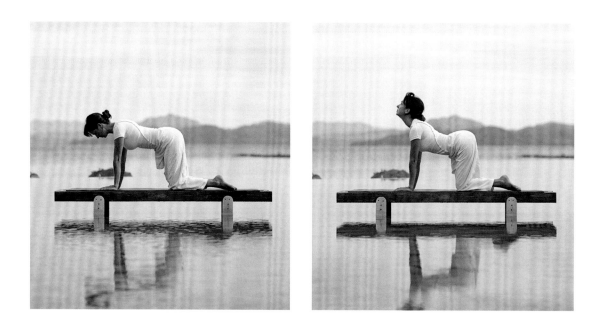

Marjaryasana/Bitilasana (Cat pose/Cow pose)

Start in a 'table-top' position with your palms under your shoulders and your knees directly under your hips and your neck in line with your torso.

As you inhale, open your belly to the earth; pointing your tailbone to the sky, open your chest through your arms and lengthen the back of your neck as you softly look up. Feel the openness of your front body.

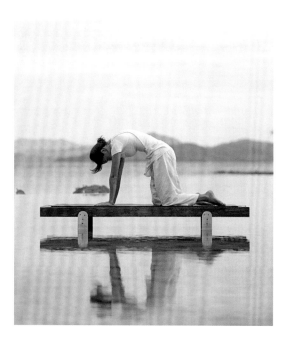

As you exhale, press your hands and knees into the floor and curl up into your chest, sternum and belly. Opening your back ribs to the sky, relax your head and hips down. Repeat the movement between these two poses 5 times, moving and breathing slowly so you can enjoy the transitions.

*top tip

These movements provide a gentle massage to the spine and belly organs and they help ease the back torso and neck. They are also beneficial for releasing stress.

Balasana
(Child's pose)

From table-top position, move into Child's Pose with your hips over your heels, arms lengthened out in front of you, forehead resting on the floor (or a cushion) and your neck and arms relaxed. Rest for 5–10 breaths.

Slide forward, back into table-top position, before moving gradually into standing.

*top tip

This pose calms the brain and helps relieve stress and fatigue. It also helps open the hips, thighs and ankles.

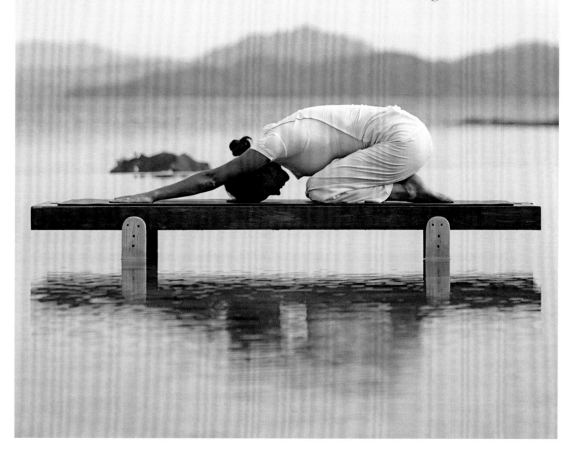

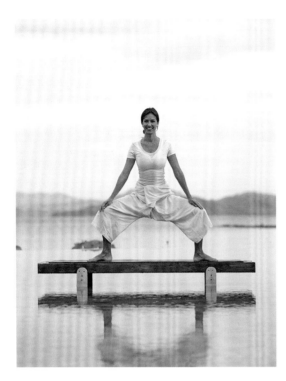

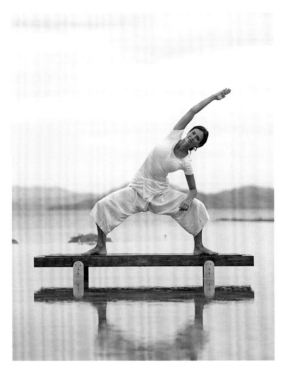

Utkata Konasana (Goddess pose)

Stand with feet a little wider than hip-width apart and toes open at a 45-degree angle, knees bent in the direction of your middle toe, thighs rotated outward, spine relaxed and tailbone pointing to the floor. Rest your hands on your thighs and soften your shoulders and upper body into the strength of your legs. Breathe evenly and softly for 5 breaths. (You may straighten your legs for a rest.)

Come back to your squat and, as you inhale, place the left elbow onto your left thigh (or place your hand, if this feels like too much). Exhale and lengthen from your right hip into your right ribs, as you open your right arm over your ear and over your head, your side opening to the sky. Breathe in this pose for 5 breaths.

Inhale back into the centre with a neutral spine and exhale, then repeat on the other side. Do this 3 times, then return to standing to rest your legs before the next pose.

*top tip

This pose strengthens and stretches the thighs, hips, groin, knees and ankles and it helps increase circulation in these areas. Side-opening helps open the waist, chest, lungs and shoulders and stimulates the abdominal organs.

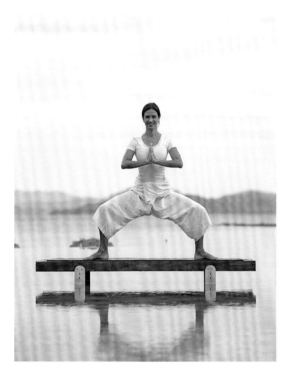

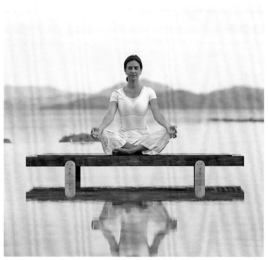

Inhale and come back to the centre in your squat, placing both palms together in front of your heart. This hand gesture is used to induce a meditative state of awareness. It is also a gesture to express reverence, honour and celebration.

As you remain in this pose, breathe into your lower body. Allow a little intensity and heat to arise in your thighs and legs. Feel the reverence in your heart, honour your body and celebrate in your heart as you welcome life (and flow) into your body and pelvis.

You can hold this pose for up to 3 minutes, but start with 1 minute and build up slowly.

At the end of your practice, come to a comfortable seated position. You can raise your hips on a cushion or a bolster and cross your feet in front of you.

Rest your hands on your legs or knees and let your index finger and thumb touch. Close your eyes and receive your breath with your belly and relax your pelvic floor as you inhale. Soften and surrender as you exhale, and release your breath and anything that it would serve you to let go of. Feel free to lie down on your back with your palms open by your sides.

*top tip
This pose increases stamina
and the circulation
of energy.

TOP TEN FOODS TO BOOST FERTILITY

Here are ten Clean & Lean foods that will help to improve and extend not only your fertility, but also that of your partner. If you're already pregnant or a mum, eat them anyway to keep you healthy and feeling great.

FOR HER...

1. Full-fat dairy: Researchers from Harvard University found women who eat at least one serving of full-fat dairy a day reduce their risk of infertility by more than a quarter. The dairy is thought to help improve ovarian function. Forget low-fat or diet yogurts as they often contain sugar to make up for the lack of fat. Instead, tuck into full-fat Greek yogurt, organic milk and quality (less-processed) cheese.

2. Olive oil: Harvard researchers found that olive and certain other oils – like flaxseed – can boost female fertility by promoting proper hormone function.

3. Folate-rich foods: Folic acid, also known as vitamin B_9, is essential for all women who are trying to conceive or in the first 12 weeks of pregnancy as it protects against neural tube defects such as spina bifida. A 400mcg supplement is recommended, together with folate-rich foods such as broccoli, spinach, asparagus and lentils.

4. Orange fruit and vegetables: The body converts orange foods that are rich in beta-carotene to vitamin A, which supports healthy ovulation.

5. Vegetarian protein: According to a study at Harvard University, women who eat more plant proteins (eg. nuts, chickpeas and legumes), are more likely to get pregnant than those who get their proteins from red meat as the latter are harder to digest and this can send hormone levels out of balance, thus affecting fertility.

6. Oily fish: The omega-3 fatty acids found in oily fish help to regulate reproductive hormones, relieve stress and increase blood flow to the sexual organs. Vegetarians can get omega-3 fatty acids from walnuts, pumpkin seeds, flaxseed oil and eggs.

FOR HIM...

1. Spinach: It's a great source of folate, which improves sperm production. A study from the University of California found that men who regularly eat spinach had up to 30 per cent healthier sperm, so eat it a couple of times a week to improve your fertility.

2. Honey: Researchers at the University of Western Australia found that the antioxidants present in honey may prevent sperm damage and increase sperm health. Pick a good-quality manuka honey, as it contains more health-boosting antioxidants than regular honey. Spread it thinly on oatcakes or fresh rye bread.

3. Brazil nuts: A study from the University of Padua showed that just three of these a day can prevent damage to sperm from environmental factors.

4. Brightly coloured fruits and vegetables: Researchers at the University of Rochester NY, USA found that brightly coloured fruits and vegetables such as tomatoes, beetroot, peppers and oranges, which contain the antioxidants glutathione and cryptoxanthin, are associated with strong, healthy sperm.

OUR COVER GIRL'S STORY

My wife Christiane gave birth to our beautiful daughter Charlotte in 2012. Here's her story.

'Being a mum is even more amazing than I ever expected. Every moment with Charlotte is heart-warming and it often feels like she's been in our lives for ever. I now know what it feels like to be completely fulfilled and content. But the road to getting pregnant was long and rocky, so we know first-hand how difficult fertility struggles can be.

'After a wonderful wedding in the summer of 2010 James and I started trying for a family immediately. As you'd expect, we're both fit and healthy; James has spent his whole career getting people into shape, and he's advised lots of female clients who were trying to conceive. So, if I'm honest, I took our fertility for granted.

'Coming from a family of healthy, fertile women I never thought I'd have any issues myself. But after James and I got married I had my contraceptive implant removed, and my period never arrived. I put it down to my body adjusting and the fact that I travelled a lot for work. But as the months went by and I still wasn't pregnant we started to worry.

'After what felt like the longest year of my life, we saw a specialist who told us, following various tests, that there was no medical reason for our inability to conceive. It wasn't a relief – it was just incredibly frustrating. At least if there was a problem we could try to fix it, but all we could do was live in an awful state of limbo and keep on hoping.

'We're positive people, but the sadness started to set in. I looked at our friends and family and everybody around us seemed to be having babies. When would it be our turn? It wasn't fair and we felt utterly powerless. I remember sitting in our gynaecologist's office in tears as he explained we might never conceive.

'But I knew in my heart that my purpose in life was to have lots of children, so I never gave in to the negative results and comments. I wanted to take some control over the situation, so with the advice of fertility experts I tweaked my diet, which was good anyway. I cut down on the amount I was exercising. (Too much exercise,

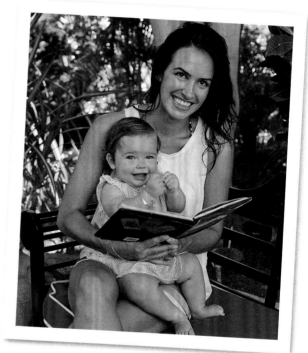

especially cardio, can put extra stress on the body and make your cycles irregular; it was making me underweight, too.) I also turned to alternative therapies like acupuncture and reflexology.

'James and I stayed positive and I kept telling myself it would happen. I still knew I was destined to be a mother, and I couldn't see a future without a child in it, so I trusted that it would happen at the right time.

'We were offered fertility-enhancing drugs, but we wanted to take a more natural route. However, as the months went on, we eventually decided to try Clomid, which is used to induce ovulation. Amazingly, though, my period arrived the day we were due to get the drug.

'Still the months went on and I wasn't pregnant. It was incredibly hard, but we used to repeat these little mantras to each other every day about how grateful we were for having each other, our friends, family and soon our little healthy baby. We decided we didn't want this struggle to make us bitter or angry. I'm not saying that it was always easy or that we never felt those emotions, but it helped us.

'Then a chance meeting with an old friend and her daughter led us to consider IVF. It's important for me to mention that we'd never had anything against IVF; we had just decided it wasn't for us at the start. But after seeing our friend's utterly beautiful baby we realised we had to go for it.

'We booked an appointment for IVF, but another coincidence was around the corner: on the day of our appointment I had a really weird feeling I was pregnant. Although my periods had returned, I was now a week late. Initially I had just put this down to my cycle being irregular, but that morning I took a pregnancy test and watched wide-eyed as the line appeared to show it was positive. Despite the fact that this was everything I'd ever dreamed of, I didn't jump for joy. I felt calm and almost detached and, looking back, I guess I didn't want to get my hopes up in case it wasn't true. I showed James the test and he was also very calm. We had a cuddle with big smiles and teary eyes and both felt quietly happy, hoping and praying this was it and that we'd finally get our baby.

'As the pregnancy progressed, I let myself relax and then I became really excited as I watched my bump grow. However, I had terrible morning sickness. I desperately wanted to eat healthily for the baby, but I was vomiting the whole time and just craved white carbs (in Chapter 8 James gives plenty of tips on dealing with cravings in a Clean & Lean way). I soon learned that my baby would take everything it needed from me to be healthy and leave me without! So I kept my vitamin supply up with a prenatal multivitamin. My energy levels were very low and I would find myself in bed all day. I was putting on weight and watching my belly grow and, as beautiful as this process is, I started feeling bad about myself. This was not what I was expecting. I had to turn these feelings around because my baby and I were now one. Anything I felt, the baby would also feel.

'I made a point of still going for walks and doing gentle yoga as this helped keep me feeling good and strong. I learned to listen to my body and do what it told me, but taking away any shame or guilt about myself or what I was doing. I learned to embrace the entire process and all the beautiful changes that my body was going through, so that my baby would grow healthy and strong inside me. One of the first of many sacrifices we make for our children! But the end result, having that baby safely in your arms, is a blissful feeling that is indescribable.

'Thankfully, my labour was straightforward and Charlotte was born weighing 7lb. It was a drug-free, natural labour with only James and the midwife in the room with me. I had done a lot of preparation for it which made me feel empowered and excited about the birth. I had visualised exactly how I wanted it to go and it went to plan. And then came Charlotte; I felt completely overwhelmed when they put her on my chest. I took in her tiny features and couldn't believe she was here at last, as I always knew she would be.

> *Now every time we look at Charlotte we are so grateful. We would have waited a lifetime for her to come into our lives.*

'Life since Charlotte's birth has been so wonderful, full of joy, love and peace. James is the most amazing, loving and supportive father and the best thing of all is that he is always there. Times are not always easy with a newborn – there is so much to learn for both mum and baby. There are many nights with broken sleep, cries when you just wish you could take away their distress, an extraordinary amount of hormones flooding through your body and energy-zapping breastfeeding.

'What really worked for us was having a routine from day one. It helps us to predict why Charlotte may be crying, and to know that she is getting enough sleep and food. All her needs are being met now, as well as mine. And when we put Charlotte to bed at 7pm and James and I have the evening to ourselves, all we do is look at pictures and watch videos of her from the day!

'I now look back on my journey and in a way I feel grateful it took so long because I now know what it means to be truly healthy. It's about eating well and mindfully (and now passing this on to Charlotte while weaning her), doing balanced exercise, using natural therapies, learning to relax through meditation, trusting in life and my body and keeping a strong and positive mind, free from shame and guilt.'

MY FAVOURITE READS

While you're trying:
✳ *The Baby-Making Bible* by Emma Cannon

During pregnancy:
✳ *What to Expect When You're Expecting* by Heidi Murkoff

Before the birth:
✳ *Effective Birth Preparation: Your Practical Guide to a Better Birth* by Maggie Howell
✳ *Birth Skills: Proven Pain Management Techniques for your Labour and Birth* by Juju Sundin

Post-baby:
✳ *The Contented Little Baby Book* by Gina Ford

Any time:
✳ *Buddhism for Mothers: A Calm Approach to Caring for Yourself and Your Children* by Sarah Napthali

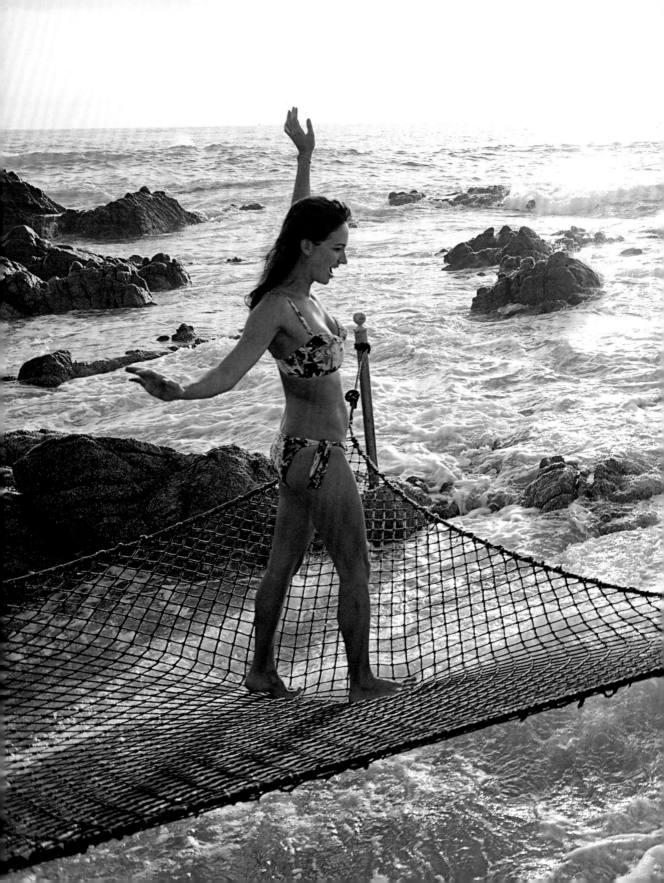

CHAPTER 3

THE FIRST TRIMESTER

WEEKS 1–12

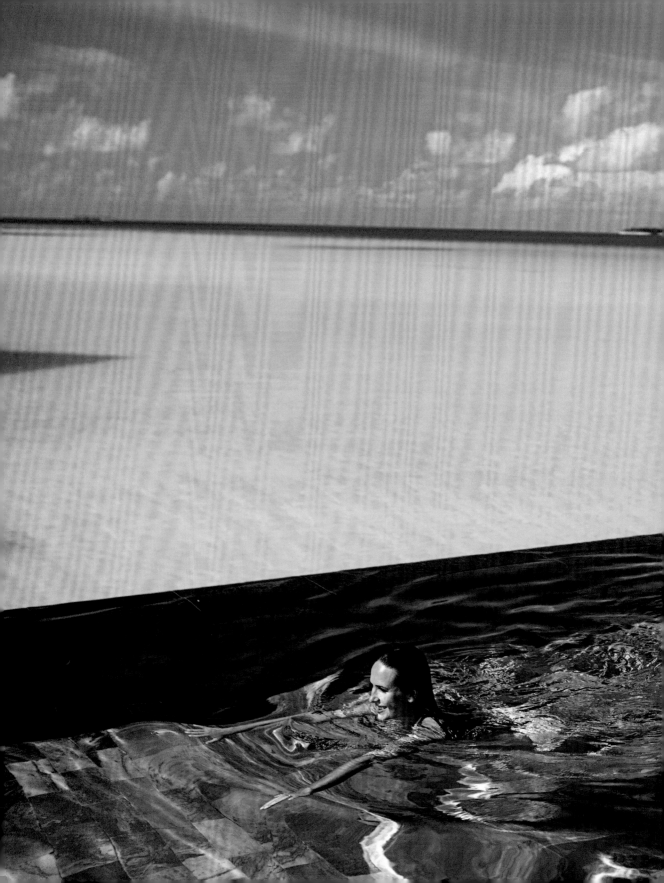

FROM THE MIDWIFE

Having a good midwife to help you through pregnancy is absolutely essential and Christiane and myself were lucky to be supported by the very best – Julie Schiller. Below, she lets you know how your baby is growing in the first trimester.

'At four weeks old, your unborn baby is a cluster of developing cells around the size of a poppy seed. The yolk sac is producing nutrients and red blood cells for your baby, and the placenta and umbilical cord are getting ready to take over. By five weeks, your baby's heart starts to beat, buds are starting to sprout that will eventually become its arms and legs, and organs are beginning to develop. The head is still disproportionately large compared to the body and by nine weeks the genitals are starting to form, although it'll be hard to determine the sex for a few more weeks. By ten weeks all the important organs – such as the brain, lungs and kidneys – are fully formed. By the end of the first trimester your baby is the size of a lime and can close its fingers and curl its toes. Your uterus, which started off the size of an orange, is now the size of a grapefruit. Much of your baby's crucial development has taken place this trimester and now it's time for it to get bigger and stronger.'
BY JULIE SCHILLER

*top tip

Listen to your body during pregnancy. Sit down and rest when your body tells you to and, if you're tired, choose sleep over exercise in this trimester.

The first trimester is often the hardest and most tiring for many women. In fact, one of the first symptoms of pregnancy for some is extreme tiredness. Nobody knows for sure why this is, but it's thought to be due to the hormonal changes that are taking place – especially the increase in the hormones progesterone and oestrogen.

The most important thing to do during these first twelve weeks of pregnancy is to listen to your body: so rest when you feel like it, and sleep whenever you can (if this is your first pregnancy, it may be the last chance you'll get for a while); and if you're hungry, eat something. It's that simple. Your body has the amazing ability to tell you exactly what it needs (so listen up), and this is truer now than ever. Nature will always do its job and help your baby grow strong and healthy, so try to relax and embrace all the changes that are coming your way.

That said, you can always tweak your lifestyle to make the first twelve weeks a little easier by eating Clean & Lean. It's one of the best things you can do for yourself and your baby, as you'll both be getting lots of lovely nutrients and avoiding empty calories and unhealthy additives and toxins. It won't always be easy in the first trimester, when you may be feeling unusually tired, hungry or sick, so try not to put too much pressure on yourself. If you follow the basics of Clean & Lean 80 per cent of the time, it won't matter if you go off track a little. Just remember, as always, to be kind to yourself.

In this chapter I'm going to give you tips and advice on staying Clean & Lean during the first trimester, along with some gentle exercises you can do if you feel up to it. They're not designed to keep you in shape (although that will be an added bonus), but to keep your body strong and supple to carry you through your pregnancy journey. And just a little reminder – you're amazing for creating another little person!

WHAT YOU MAY BE EXPERIENCING RIGHT NOW

Morning sickness

This can often be one of the worst first-trimester symptoms and it affects three quarters of pregnant women. Despite its name, it can occur at any time of the day (or even all day). However, most women experience it in the first half of the day – most likely because they haven't eaten overnight (while they've slept). Experts agree that hormonal changes are the cause of morning sickness.

What to do: One of the best ways to combat it is to keep your blood-sugar levels steady and you can do this by eating Clean & Lean. Eat five small meals a day, which roughly translates as three meals plus a couple of snacks in between. However, keep your meals smaller and your snacks bigger than usual so all five 'meals' are approximately the same size.

If you're craving carbohydrates, go for energy-boosting ones like oats, spelt, brown rice and quinoa. If you crave sugar, have some, but don't go overboard. Sugary foods actually make you more tired in the long run – they give you a hit of energy when you eat them because they cause a massive spike in your blood-sugar levels, but this is followed by a crash, which leaves you tired and craving more sugar. Instead, eat Clean & Lean foods, little and often, and keep treats for the odd occasion when you really fancy them.

Swollen, tender breasts

Hormonal surges in the first trimester can make your breasts feel swollen and tender. It isn't milk, which comes along just before you give birth and in the days afterwards.

What to do: This usually settles down after the second trimester but it's a good idea to go for a bra fitting in your first trimester to make sure you're wearing the right size.

TIPS FOR COPING WITH MORNING SICKNESS

✳ Keep a supply of oatcakes by your bed, so if you wake up hungry in the night or first thing in the morning you can munch on them.

✳ Avoid drinking fluids for fifteen minutes before and after meals, and never during mealtimes. Your digestion slows down in pregnancy and drinking fluids slows it down even further. So stay hydrated (see p. 61), but avoid drinking too close to mealtimes.

✳ Don't overdo it – sleep when you're tired, and this will really help with the sickness.

✳ Try ginger – have a cup of ginger tea (see p. 18) or use it ground in your food.

✳ Minimise stress – easier said than done, but try to avoid stressful situations as it's thought stress makes nausea worse.

✳ Try acupuncture or reflexology – find pregnancy-specific experts local to you.

✳ Accept it – if nothing else works, just remember it's a phase. It will pass. I promise!

Excess saliva

Excess saliva in early pregnancy is called ptyalism and it's completely harmless for you and your baby. Doctors don't really know what causes it although, like many pregnancy symptoms, it's thought to be due to changing hormones. **What to do:** Brush your teeth regularly, drink plenty of water, eat small and frequent meals and avoid starchy foods like bread and potatoes.

Frequent need to urinate

This is another of the first symptoms for many women and it usually starts at around six weeks after conception (and often gets more pronounced with each pregnancy). You can blame your hormones again – they cause more blood flow to your kidneys, so your bladder fills up more quickly. The amount of blood flow in your body rises throughout your pregnancy too, meaning your kidneys also have to process more fluid. Then, as your baby grows, it starts to put more pressure on your bladder. Don't worry, though – apart from being annoying, it's perfectly harmless. **What to do:** Don't be tempted to drink less to avoid too many bathroom trips, as it's important to stay hydrated (in a nutshell, this ensures nutrients from your food are delivered to your baby). However, as long as you've drunk enough in the day it's fine to cut back on water before bedtime to avoid nocturnal bathroom visits. Avoid or cut down on diuretics like tea and coffee, and make sure you fully empty your bladder each time you pee by leaning slightly forward towards the end. Lastly, don't try to hold it in or delay bathroom trips, as this makes the problem worse and could even lead to a UTI (urinary tract infection).

Bleeding gums

The hormone progesterone increases blood flow to the gums, so you may notice you get bleeding gums, especially after brushing your teeth. **What to do:** This should rectify itself after you give birth, but in the meantime brush and floss regularly and gently. If it gets particularly bad, you should see a dentist.

Bloating and gas

Blame those hormones again. Progesterone relaxes the tissue in your gastrointestinal tract, which slows down your digestion, causing gas and bloating. **What to do:** Eat little and often, chew your food thoroughly (at least fifteen times per mouthful) and try not

to drink during meals. And have a sense of humour about it Christiane and I found the huge truck driver farts hilarious (she'll love me for telling you that).

Leg cramps

Your already-growing uterus can put pressure on one of the main veins from your legs, creating circulation problems. As you gain weight during pregnancy, the pressure gets worse. Leg cramps can also indicate a nutrient deficiency, such as calcium or magnesium. **What to do:** Drink plenty of fluids and avoid sitting or standing up for long periods. Do simple exercises such as rotating your foot and stretching your calves.

Constipation

Like bloating and gas, this is due to hormonal changes slowing down the digestive tract. It can feel particularly uncomfortable when your baby gets bigger. **What to do:** Drink plenty of water and eat fibre-rich foods, which will also keep your bowels healthy and regular (so helping to prevent haemorrhoids and piles). Gentle exercise helps too, as does a glass of warm water (boil it and wait for it to cool down) with a slice of lemon first thing in the morning to flush out your system.

Food aversions
and cravings

Have you suddenly gone off your favourite foods? You're not alone – 85 per cent of women experience food aversions in early pregnancy (Christiane went off most foods for her entire pregnancy). As for cravings, they're often your body's way of telling you what it needs. **What to do:** Many women go off meat protein, so if this is you, try to include some vegetarian protein in your diet instead in the form of beans and pulses (do I hear someone say gas'?). Don't worry too much – food aversions usually go by the second trimester and there are tips for handling cravings in Chapter 8.

Reflux and heartburn

In pregnancy, the hormone progesterone relaxes the valve that separates the oesophagus (gullet) and the stomach and this allows stomach acid to come up, causing an uncomfortable burning sensation in the back of the throat. It's made worse by the fact that your digestion is slower and increases as the baby grows and pushes your stomach upwards, shortening your oesophagus.

What to do: Avoid fizzy drinks and alcohol, caffeine, sugary, fatty or spicy foods and citrus fruits. Don't eat big meals – eat several small ones instead (and not too close to bedtime) – and chew thoroughly. Wear loose clothes that aren't tight around your chest, ribcage or stomach. At night, when it's often worse, prop yourself up using pillows and speak to your doctor or midwife if it's particularly bad as they may prescribe medication.

Irritability

Did you expect you'd feel on top of the world, but find instead that every little thing is annoying you? Don't worry, it's perfectly normal and all down to fluctuating hormones. I just want to share a brilliant story about Christiane here: when she was expecting Charlotte, she told me off for breathing in an annoying way. I asked her if perhaps her hormones were making her grumpy, and she said: 'No, you've just become more annoying since I became pregnant.' We laugh about it now, but I'm pretty sure she meant it at the time.

What to do: Try to talk about your concerns to your partner, friends, family or midwife. Find ways to relax, such as meditation, which will also boost your mood. And if you do feel particularly low and are crying most days, see your doctor or midwife, as it could be a sign of depression.

Dry or spotty skin

Some women find their skin gets drier, more oily or spotty. And yes – it's those pregnancy hormones yet again.

What to do: Eat Clean & Lean with plenty of skin-loving foods like salmon, vegetables, fruits and nuts. Cleanse your skin thoroughly (though gently) and drink lots of water. By the third trimester any skin problems should clear up. But, as always, don't worry if they don't. Remember that what is happening is amazing and so are you.

Breathlessness

This is very common in pregnancy. Hormonal changes cause you to breathe more deeply, which can feel like breathlessness. As your baby gets bigger it also puts pressure on your lungs, reducing their capacity, so you get out of breath more easily.

What to do: This goes once you've given birth, but in the meantime, take it easy and don't push yourself too hard.

Snoring

Higher levels of the hormone oestrogen can cause a swelling in the nose lining which can lead to snoring. Increased blood flow also causes a swelling in the nose and excessive weight gain can make the problem worse.

What to do: Try to stick to the recommended weight gain during your pregnancy and sleep on your left side.

ON THE PLUS SIDE...

It's not all bad news: as well as experiencing some unpleasant pregnancy symptoms, you may also be discovering some definite perks!

SHINY, THICK HAIR

During pregnancy your hair may look thicker, bouncier and more shiny. It's not that you're growing any more hair – just that you're not losing any; you may well have noticed that it's not falling out during hair washes or brushing. An increased blood flow to the scalp can also result in shinier locks.

GLOWING SKIN

Increased blood flow brings more blood to the face, giving you a smoother complexion. Plus, if you cut out alcohol (which should be a pregnancy given) and sugary foods, your skin will glow even more.

FULLER BREASTS

Even before your milk comes in your breasts may look fuller and firmer and you can go up a cup size or two.

STRONG NAILS

Hormone changes will make your nails grow faster and stronger.

STAYING SAFE THROUGHOUT YOUR PREGNANCY

You'll be bombarded with advice in your pregnancy, some true some not so true. Here's everything you need to know. And if you're unsure about anything, speak to your midwife or doctor.

Hot tubs, saunas and steam rooms: Some studies suggest that water at over 100°C can be damaging to developing cells. This is especially true in the first trimester. Becoming too hot can also slow down blood flow to the baby because blood flows to the surface of the skin instead to cool you down. You're also more likely to become dehydrated. So avoid hot tubs, saunas and steam rooms throughout your whole pregnancy and make sure your baths at home aren't too hot either.

Cats: There is often some confusion about cats and pregnancy. In a nutshell, it's perfectly safe to be around cats as long as you follow a few guidelines. Toxoplasmosis is caused by a parasite called *Toxoplasma gondii* that can be found in cat faeces (as well as in undercooked meat and sheep). If you develop toxoplasmosis in pregnancy, it can be harmful to your baby and increase your risk of miscarriage and stillbirth. However, it's important to note that this is very rare. Avoid emptying cat-litter trays and wear rubber gloves if you do. Also wear gloves while gardening (to avoid cat faeces), avoid sheep and wash your hands thoroughly if you touch a cat or a sheep.

Cleaning products: Relatively little is known about the effects of cleaning products on pregnant women; however, I'd advise you to err on the side of caution because your baby absorbs what you absorb. Avoid big jobs like cleaning the oven, as oven cleaners let off a lot of fumes. If you do use products like cleaning sprays and air fresheners, keep the windows open so air circulates. Better still, opt for a natural cleaning product that doesn't use chemicals. For example, a company I love called e-cloth makes cloths in which microfibres trap dirt and grime using just water, without any need for chemical cleaners. They're great for you (they've been approved by Allergy UK) and the environment, as you're not flushing cleaning chemicals down the bath or sink.

Paint fumes: Before the 1970s, lead elements were found in paint which were shown to be harmful to unborn babies. Although the risks from popular household paints today are very low, why take the chance? Don't schedule decorating during your pregnancy and, if you do, stay away from the paint and keep doors and windows open. Also avoid eating, drinking or sleeping in a room that's recently been painted.

Pollution: A 2013 study from the Harvard School of Public Health found that pregnant women exposed to high levels of pollution were up to twice as likely to have a child with autism. However, it's important to remember that they were exposed to high levels. Walking along a busy road won't do you any harm and millions of women who live in big, smoky cities have healthy babies. However, it's worth trying to avoid pollution where possible – so if you walk to work along a busy road, switch to a greener route if you can.

Smoking: If you're currently pregnant, I'm sure you don't smoke; the fact that you're reading this book means that you care about your health and that of your baby, but I want to cover everything here, so this is a quick reminder that it's absolutely not OK – ever – to smoke during pregnancy. Anything that you eat, drink or inhale gets into your baby's bloodstream, including cigarette smoke, which contains thousands of chemicals, many of which can cause cancer. Nicotine and carbon monoxide are two of the most harmful chemicals and can cause miscarriage, premature birth and low birthweight. Nicotine also reduces your baby's oxygen supply and studies have found that babies whose mothers smoked during pregnancy are more likely to have a heart defect and lungs that do not develop properly, and there is also more chance that they will have a low IQ, behavioural problems and developmental delays. Plus, smoking can reduce your fertility by 40 per cent, so if you are trying to conceive, quit as soon as possible.

If you're struggling to give up smoking, speak to your GP or midwife immediately and ask them for information on how to quit, including courses and self-help techniques. Now is the time to focus on your own and your baby's health. You both deserve a happy, healthy life.

C&L FOODS FOR PREGNANCY

IT'S WORTH REMEMBERING:

✳ You need to cook fish, meat and poultry thoroughly, so they're piping hot throughout with no trace of pink or blood.

✳ Cook your eggs well, so the white and yolk are solid. For this reason it's better to have scrambled eggs or omelettes, rather than poached eggs which can be runny.

✳ Be extra vigilant about washing fruits and vegetables.

✳ Have only pasteurised milk, yogurt and cheese.

✳ Take a 400 mcg supplement of folic acid for the first 12 weeks of pregnancy, and a 10mcg supplement of vitamin D throughout pregnancy and breastfeeding

✳ Limit yourself to two portions of oily fish a week. They can contain high levels of mercury, which can be harmful to your baby's developing nervous system.

AND AVOID THE FOLLOWING:

✳ Pâtés – whether fish, meat or vegetable, they are more likely than other foods to contain listeria bacteria, which cause listeriosis (a type of food poisoning) and you're more susceptible to it when you're pregnant because your immune system is weaker. Listeriosis is usually a mild illness, but it can harm your baby and cause premature birth and even miscarriage – it's very rare, but why take the risk?

✳ Mould-ripened soft cheese, such as brie and camembert, and blue-veined cheeses such as Danish blue and gorgonzola – they're also more likely to contain listeria.

✳ Foods containing raw or undercooked eggs, like fresh mayonnaise; shop-bought is fine as it's pasteurised.

✳ Marlin, swordfish or shark, as they contain high levels of mercury.

✳ Raw shellfish, such as oysters or mussels, because they can contain bacteria which may cause food poisoning.

✳ Liver and liver products – they contain a lot of vitamin A, which can harm a developing baby. For the same reason, don't take fish liver oil or other supplements that contain vitamin A.

FOODS YOU CAN EAT DURING PREGNANCY:

✳ Sushi – it's fine to eat sushi made with raw fish, as long as the fish used to make it has been frozen first. Raw fish can contain parasitic worms that could cause food poisoning, but freezing kills them. So buy sushi from well-established restaurant chains and ask them if their fish has been frozen. You can also opt for vegetarian sushi.

✳ Peanuts – peanuts and peanut butter are fine, as long as you don't have a nut allergy.

✳ Hard cheeses, like Cheddar and Parmesan.

✳ Soft cheeses – as long as they're made from pasteurised milk (check the label), it's safe to eat cream cheese, goat's cheese, mozzarella and halloumi.

ALWAYS KEEP THESE IN YOUR HOME:

Fresh fruit – you can grab a piece whenever you feel hungry, rather than heading for the biscuit tin.

A lemon – squeeze it over salads to add flavour or add a slice to cold water for a refreshing drink, or to warm water (boiled and then cooled) to flush out your system.

A bag of unsalted nuts – grab a handful to keep you going when you haven't had time to cook.

Avocados – the perfect snack, full of healthy, filling fats; and the creamy texture will satisfy a sweet tooth. Slice half of one over some oatcakes.

Eggs – two scrambled eggs on rye bread or an omelette filled with whatever vegetables you have in your fridge make a nutritious, filling meal, whether it's breakfast or dinner.

Something green – always try to have something green with all your meals, such as avocado, green pepper, green apples, spinach, rocket or broccoli.

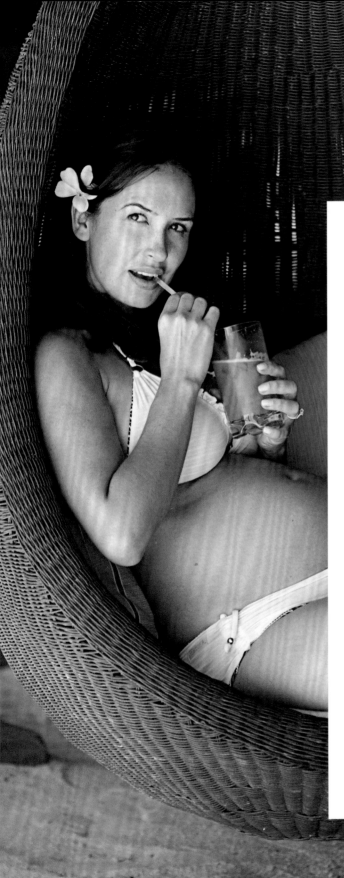

HYDRATION IN PREGNANCY

In all my Clean & Lean books I talk about good hydration, but drinking enough water is even more important in pregnancy. First, it helps deliver all the goodness from your food to your baby (and you!). Water helps your body to absorb vitamins and minerals from food and transports them to your blood cells, from where your baby laps them up, via the placenta. Water also encourages good digestion, which can slow down in pregnancy (hence why you often get constipated), and it flushes you out and takes away toxins, leaving you feeling less uncomfortable, especially as your baby grows bigger and your stomach gets squashed.

Lastly, during pregnancy you're more prone to water retention. Known as oedema, it's responsible for those pesky, puffy ankles and the fact that your rings may not fit on your fingers any more. Ironically, drinking more water helps with water retention, as it flushes you out.

And note that new mums also need to drink plenty of water for all the reasons above.

You don't need to drink more water than usual when pregnant, but you do need to make sure you drink enough. Stick to around 2 litres a day. Keep it still and filtered and avoid sugary drinks and too much caffeine which acts as a diuretic (meaning it makes you wee a lot), which can dehydrate you. Try adding lemon or cucumber slices to water. Lemon acts as a great natural detoxer and cucumber gives you a hit of vitamins (you may have noticed lots of spas add cucumber slices to their water), plus it tastes great. Or try some fresh mint leaves to help your digestion.

EXERCISE DURING PREGNANCY

If your pregnancy is normal and you feel fine and up to it, moderate exercise at this stage can help you feel better, but don't feel pressured. Just being active and walking every day is also fine.

There are several benefits of exercise during pregnancy. It can:
* ease or prevent back pain and other discomforts (as long as you do it correctly – and in this book I'll show you how)
* boost your mood and energy levels
* help you sleep better
* help prevent excess weight gain – you shouldn't be worrying about your weight in pregnancy, but nor do you need to be gaining an excessive amount
* increase stamina and muscle strength
* help prevent orthopaedic issues, such as back and knee pain
* reduce the risk of pre- and postnatal depression
* make giving birth easier
* improve your ability to deal with labour – the fitter you are, the better you'll be able to cope (trust me, this will come in handy)
* help reduce constipation, which is a common pregnancy side effect, plus it reduces swelling and bloating
* possibly prevent or help gestational diabetes. Diabetes UK agrees that it helps levels of glucose tolerance.

However, as with everything else pregnancy-related, listen to your body at all times and check with your health practitioner or midwife before exercising. If you feel unwell, breathless or as if you can't carry on at any point, stop immediately. Don't push yourself.

It's best to continue exercising in a similar manner to the way you did before you got pregnant. For example, if you ran regularly and went to the gym every week, continue with this, but listen to your body and slow things down if you need to.

If you rarely exercised before you got pregnant, don't take it up now in the hope of keeping your weight down. Instead, start slowly with walking and swimming and find a local yoga or Pilates class that specialises in pregnancy.

Stop any risky or high-impact sports, such as horse riding, road cycling (a stationary exercise bike is fine), hockey, tennis, scuba diving, skiing, ice skating or hiking at high altitudes.

Stop exercising immediately if you experience any of the following (and if the symptoms don't pass, call the maternity unit at your hospital or your doctor):
* feeling faint or dizziness
* increased shortness of breath
* chest pain
* headache
* muscle weakness
* calf pain or swelling

If any of the following happen, call the maternity unit at your hospital or your doctor immediately:
* contractions, even if they're mild and irregular
* vaginal bleeding
* decreased foetal movement in the later stages of pregnancy (you usually feel your baby's first movements at around weeks 17 or 18, though sometimes earlier with second or third pregnancies)
* fluid leaking from the vagina

TOP TIPS FOR EXERCISE DURING PREGNANCY

✳ Avoid brisk exercise in hot, humid weather.

✳ Wear comfortable clothing that will help you to remain cool.

✳ Wear a non-underwired bra that fits well and gives lots of support. It's a good idea to have your bra size professionally measured two or three times during pregnancy to ensure that you're wearing a bra that protects your growing breasts.

✳ Drink plenty of water to keep you hydrated (see p. 61).

✳ Monitor your heart rate; aim to keep it no higher than 140bpm.

✳ Stop any time you feel as though you can't go on. Remember, listen to your body.

EXERCISE IN THE FIRST TRIMESTER:

Perform the workout below 3–4 times a week on non-consecutive days. On the days between your workouts, go for a brisk walk or a light swim. Your workouts should last no longer than 30–45 minutes and, as always, ensure that you listen to your body and take plenty of rest between sets.

Perform each exercise, one after the other, until you have performed all the exercises in the circuit, then rest for 60 seconds. Between each exercise, take 30–60 seconds rest, depending on how you are feeling. Perform the whole circuit of exercises 2–3 times.

EXERCISE	REPS	SETS	REST
Tummy vacuum	8–10	2–3	30–60 secs
Hip extension	15	2–3	30–60 secs
Side-lying single-leg knee-raise with mini band	8–10/side	2–3	30–60 secs
Mini-band walking	10 steps/side	2–3	30–60 secs
Y	10–15	2–3	30–60 secs
Squat	12–15	2–3	30–60 secs
T	15	2–3	30–60 secs
Superman	12–15/side	2–3	60 secs
Hip abduction	12–15/side	2–3	60 secs

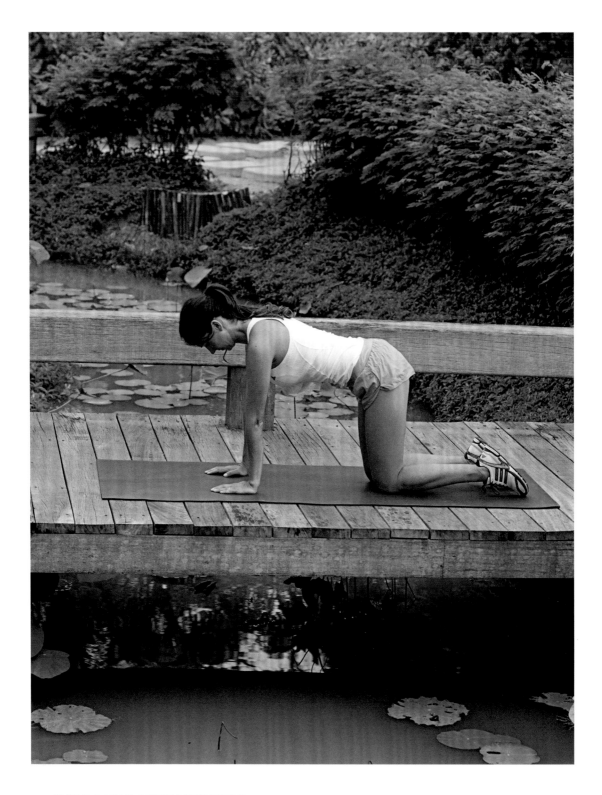

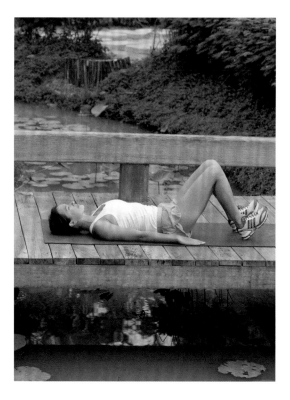 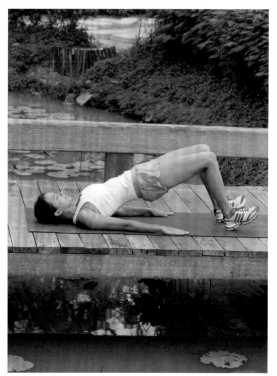

Hip extension

Start position: Lie on your back with both knees bent and heels on the ground. Point your toes up to the ceiling and place your arms by your sides.

The movement: Lift your hips off the ground, raising them as high as you can go, squeezing the glutes (your butt muscles, which help protect your lower back). Pause at the top for 1 second, then return to the start position. Repeat 15 times.

Opposite:

Tummy vacuum

Start position: Support yourself on your hands and knees with hands under shoulders, arms straight and knees under hips. Ensure your arms and thighs remain at right angles to the floor, keep your back straight and your head aligned with your upper back.

The movement: Relax your stomach, letting it sag towards the floor while maintaining a flat back. Then squeeze your tummy muscles and pull your belly button towards the ceiling, still maintaining a flat back. Repeat 8–10 times.

*top tip

This is great for your bottom and lower back. Place a Bodyism mini-band (bodyism.com) around your legs, just above your knees, for added resistance!

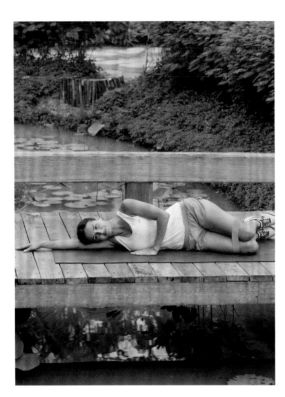

Side-lying single-leg knee-raise with mini-band

Start position: Place a Bodyism mini-band around both legs just above your knees. Lie on your right side with your right arm extended, palm facing down, and rest your head on your arm. Bend your knees to a 90-degree angle and stack them on top of one another. Keep your body in line and engage your core by pulling your belly button in towards your spine.

The movement: Raise your top knee by pushing against the resistance of the mini band. Take the knee up as far as you can without straining the lower back, keeping both feet together. With control, slowly lower back to the start position. Repeat 8–10 times on each side.

*top tip

Ensure your head is supported to create the most comfortable position for your body to be in, as well as maintaining good posture.

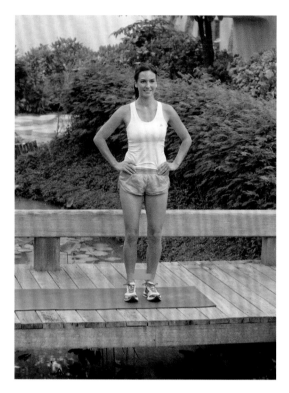
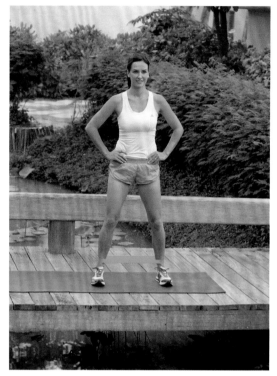

Mini-band walking

Start position: Take a Bodyism mini-band of your chosen strength and place it just above your ankles. Stand with your feet hip-width apart, hands resting on your hips and engage the core by pulling your belly button in towards your spine.

The movement: Take one large step out sideways to the right, keeping the legs straight and without using your body for momentum. Then bring your left foot in half a step, keeping tension in the band all the time. Repeat this movement for 10 steps on each side.

*top tip
This exercise strengthens and lifts your bottom like nothing else. It will also ensure your lower back stays strong and healthy throughout your pregnancy.

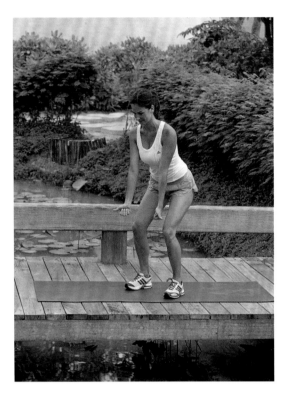
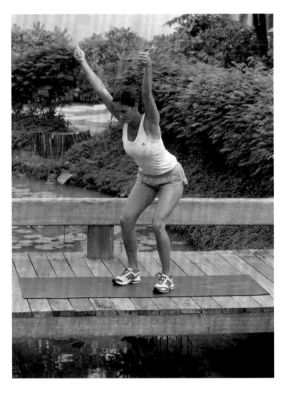

Y

Start position: Stand with your feet hip-width apart, bend your knees and stick your bottom out, so your upper body leans forward 45 degrees. Hold your hands directly below your chest with fists clenched and thumbs up, keeping your head and back all in a straight line, your shoulders back and down. Engage your core by pulling your belly button in towards the spine.

The movement: Raise both hands to create a 'Y' shape above your head with your arms by your ears, then return to the starting point. Repeat 10–15 times.

*top tip

This exercise will strengthen your shoulders and upper back. Perform the movement slowly to ensure your posture remains good throughout your pregnancy.

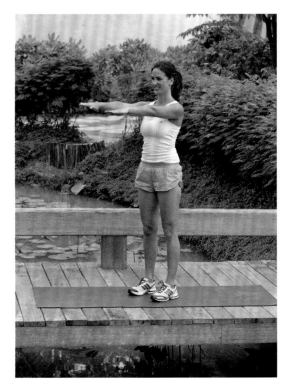
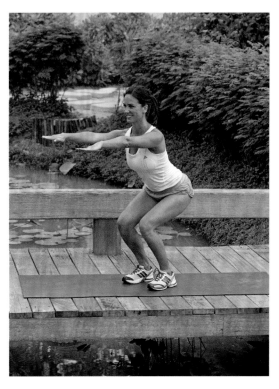

Squat

Start position: Take a comfortable stance with your feet shoulder-width apart, toes pointing forward and arms out in front of you, level with your chest. Engage your core by pulling your belly button in towards the spine.

The movement: Initiate the squat by bending the knees and by pushing the hips back. Squat back and down until the thighs are parallel to the floor. Keep your arms straight. Return to the standing position by pushing through the heels. Do not let the knees collapse inwards during the movement, keep the arms extended in front of your chest and keep your chest up and your back flat. Repeat 12–15 times.

*top tip

This is a great lower-body toner which improves balance and energy flow. It helps relax the pelvic-floor muscles, creating more room in the pelvis which can, in turn, make pregnancy, labour and childbirth more comfortable.

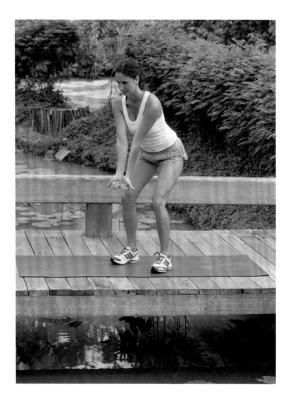
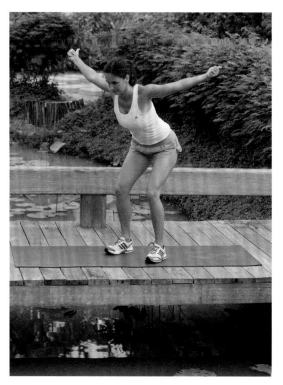

T

Start position: Stand with your feet hip-width apart. Bend your knees and lean forward so your torso is at a 45-degree angle. Keep your head and back all in a straight line, your shoulders back and down and your hands directly below your chest with fists clenched and thumbs pointing outward. Engage your core by pulling your belly button in towards the spine.

The movement: Keeping your body still and your core engaged, raise your arms out to the sides to form a 'T' shape, then return to the start position. Repeat 15 times.

*top tip
This exercise will strengthen your upper back – perfect if you have found your posture deteriorating during your pregnancy.

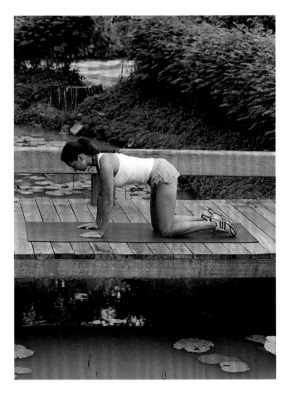
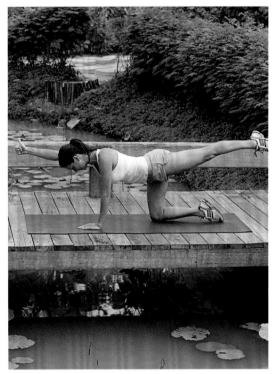

Superman

Start position: Support yourself on your hands and knees with hands under shoulders and knees under hips and with your toes firmly pointed into the floor. Ensure your spine and neck are in a straight line by keeping your gaze to the floor, just in front of your fingertips.

The movement: Extend your right arm out in front of you beyond your head, thumb up, while extending your left leg backward – imagine you are being pulled from either end. Return to the start position and repeat 12–15 times on each side.

*top tip

This exercise will activate and strengthen your hamstrings, glutes and lower-back muscles, as well as improving your overall body balance. It is also one of the safest movements to help strengthen your back throughout your pregnancy.

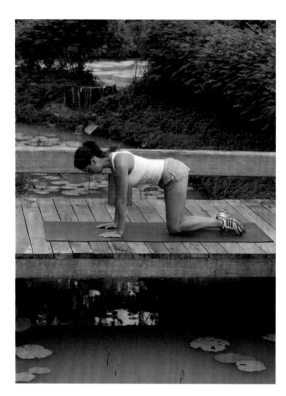 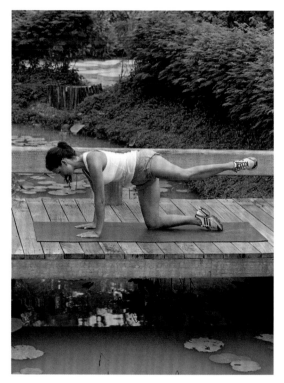

Hip abduction

Start position: Support yourself on all fours with hands under shoulders and knees under hips. Ensure your arms and thighs remain at right angles to the floor, keeping your back straight and your head aligned with your upper back. Draw your bellybutton in towards your spine to engage the core.

The movement: Keeping your upper body still – a flat back and straight arms – slowly lift your left knee to the side and slightly back, whilst keeping the knee bent throughout the movement. Then slowly return to the start position and repeat 12–15 times before moving on to the opposite leg.

*top tip

This exercise is great for strengthening and toning the glutes (your butt muscles, which help protect your lower back). Perform the movement slowly and keep your breathing regular to ensure your body stays calm and not stressed.

YOGA FOR PREGNANCY

Wenche Beard is an amazing lady and yoga expert who we've worked with for years. She designed a brilliant programme that nurtured Christiane throughout her pregnancy and I'm so happy she is able to share her wisdom here. Wenche says:

'Pregnancy is a magical experience and you should celebrate the life growing inside you. When you're pregnant and practising yoga, it gives you the opportunity to connect with your changing body and your growing baby. In the busy-ness of life, mums-to-be need some time to stop and connect with themselves in a deeper way.

'During pregnancy your body goes through some tremendous changes as it evolves to accommodate your growing baby. In my experience of working with pregnant women, I've found that they should practise yoga asanas [postures] to stay strong and in the best possible shape.

'Yoga won't just give you a healthy body, but a healthy mind too, helping you to balance your emotions through the hormonal and physical changes that are taking place. Yoga asanas and pranayama [breath control] can help prevent common pregnancy ailments such as sickness, shortness of breath, heartburn, swollen ankles and sciatica. It also helps you prepare for the birth as it enables you to "tune in" to your body and assists with better breathing techniques. Before practising yoga in pregnancy, always consult your prenatal health-care provider, doctor or midwife for advice.

'When you practice yoga in pregnancy you practise yoga with your baby at the very centre of your body and your baby will always from now on be at the very centre of your life. *Namaste*.'

BY WENCHE BEARD, British Wheel of Yoga teacher (BWY)

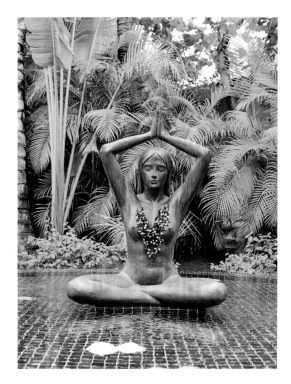

*top tip

If you are going to do yoga during pregnancy, please be careful to make sure your instructor is qualified for pregnancy yoga. Get references and follow your instincts.

Yoga moves for your first trimester

'Major changes are taking place during these first three months of your pregnancy. This is the trimester where your foetus is implanting itself into your uterus. And even though it's tiny, already at ten weeks your little one is wriggling and moving about even though you won't be able to feel it for several more weeks yet.

'I'm often asked, "Should I practise yoga in the first trimester?" If you're a healthy and active woman, and you've been practising yoga for a while, the answer is yes, though you may want to adjust your routine slightly. If you're new to yoga, it's often recommended to wait until you're twelve weeks pregnant before starting. I always recommend that clients speak to their health-care provider or doctor as soon as they discover they're pregnant for advice on exercise. In most cases your doctor will be happy for you to get on to the yoga mat.'

HERE ARE WENCHE'S YOGA-IN-PREGNANCY PRECAUTIONS:

✳ Avoid stretching your muscles too much, especially your stomach muscles.
✳ Take care in standing poses as gravity and balance change. Use supports such as blocks, walls or sturdy tables.
✳ Avoid deep belly twists.
✳ Avoid deep back bends.
✳ Avoid sharp movements.
✳ Avoid holding asanas (postures) for too long.
✳ Listen to your body at all times and stop if you feel uncomfortable.

Breathing/pranayama

'Pranayama, the "yogic breath", is a deeper, more controlled breath. "Prana" means energy and "ayama" means distributing energy. When we breathe in, we inhale oxygen and prana (life energy); this is vital for the functioning of your body and the healthy growth of your baby. As we breathe out, we release carbon dioxide and other impurities the body doesn't need. The breath is a vital part of life, and when you are breathing well, your baby is breathing well too.'

The breath control

'Get comfortable in a seated position, keeping your arms relaxed and your hands resting in your lap. Or in the "gyan mudra" (where your arms are straight, with the back of your hands on your knees and your index finger and thumb touching – this is the most common hand position in meditation and some pranayama practices). Or keep your hands on your abdomen, cradling your baby and feeling the rise and fall of your belly as you breathe. The breathing technique is known as Ujjayi breathing, and is often referred to as the "ocean breath", because the sound at the back of the throat resembles that of the ocean. When you practise this breath, there is a slight contraction of the vocal cords as you breathe in and out through the nose deeply, keeping your jaw, face, shoulders and belly relaxed. Breathe in fully and exhale completely, drinking the life force available to you and your baby, oxygenating your blood flow, making your blood purer, strengthening your lungs, enhancing your energy levels, balancing your nervous system and creating a sense of better wellbeing.

'The simple technique of Ujjayi breathing can also help during the physical and emotional demands of labour and birth. When you're fearful or in pain, your body produces the stress hormone adrenaline and produces less of the feel-good hormone oxytocin, which facilitates birth and makes labour progress. The more relaxed your body is, the easier the birth.'

Opposite are some moves to begin with.

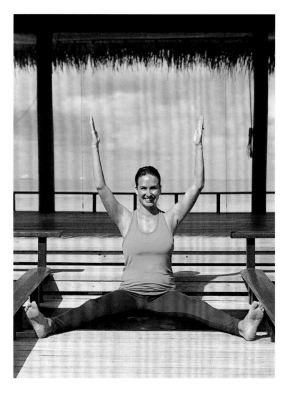

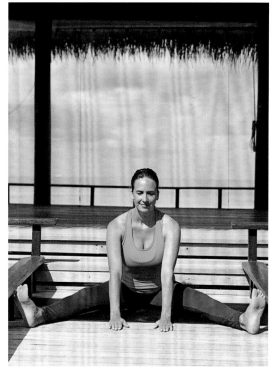

Upavistha Konasana (Wide-angle seated forward bend)

Sit on the floor with your legs as wide apart as you can comfortably get them. Tilt your pelvis, so that you sit on your 'sitting bones'.

Let the spine rise from the floor, and move the top of your head towards the sky. Lift your arms above your head, so your fingers face the sky as you inhale.

As you exhale, extend the body forward into the forward bend, lengthening the torso. Bring your hands on to the floor and relax your shoulders. Stay for 6–9 healthy breaths.

*top tip

This is a gentle stretch for the hips and lower back, which can become tight during pregnancy. Remember that it's important you don't strain yourself, so stretch only as far as is comfortable and keep movements relaxed and fluid.

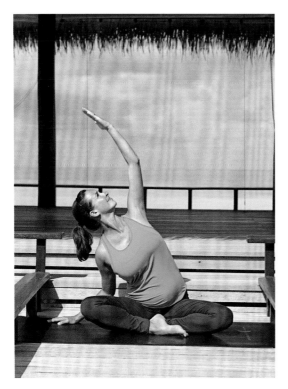

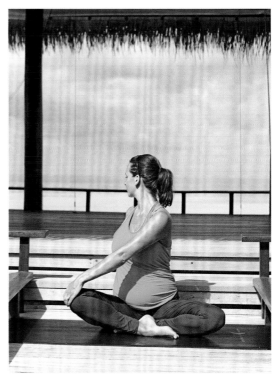

Sukhasana side stretch (Easy pose side stretch)

Sit cross-legged on the floor (or with your legs wide, if you prefer) with your arms by your sides.

Practise a long spine and place your right hand on the floor. As you inhale, let the left hand rise to the sky along the left side of the body.

As you exhale, slowly lean over to the right side and lift and rotate your upper chest, gazing upwards at the sky. Stay for 3–6 breaths, breathing into the left side of your body. Come back to the centre on an inhale and repeat on the other side.

Sukhasana twist (Cross-legged seated upper-spinal twist)

Sit cross-legged on the floor (or with your legs wide, if you prefer), with your spine tall; place your left hand on your right knee and rest the right hand on the floor behind you.

Inhale through the length of your spine, then exhale and let the exhalation take you into this gentle upper spinal twist. Stay for 3–6 breaths, keeping the crown of your head high to the sky and your chest wide.

Come back to the centre on an inhale. Exhale, digesting the benefits before repeating on the other side.

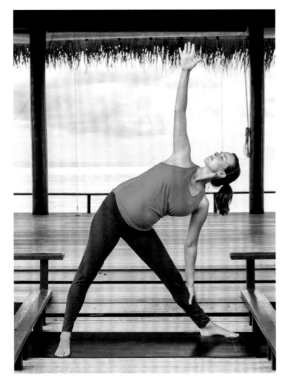

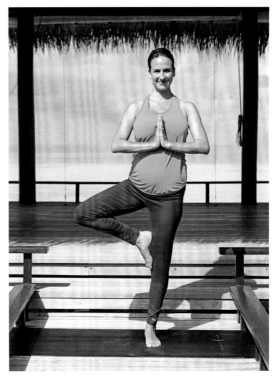

Trikonasana (Triangle pose)

Stand tall, aware of your baby at the very centre of your body, then walk your feet about a metre or so apart. Place your hands on your hips and turn your right foot 90 degrees, aligning your right heel with your left instep, hips level to the front.

Drop your arms by the side of your body and, as you inhale, lift the arms out to the side, parallel to the floor. Then, as you exhale, draw back through the left hip as you extend your torso over your left leg with an open waist. (Support yourself on your leg, blocks or even a chair if you need to.) Reach up to the sky with your right arm, keeping your neck long and remembering your head is an extension of the spine.

Lengthen the tailbone towards your right heel, keep the legs strong, the spine long and arms active. Stay for 3–6 breaths, then come back on an inhale and lower the arms on the exhale. Take a few breaths here with your hands on your belly, embodying the state of balance for both you and your baby. Repeat on the other side.

Vrksasana (Tree pose)

Stand tall, imagining roots growing into the earth from the base of your feet, like a tree. Transfer weight into the left foot and lift the right leg, placing the foot, toes pointing down, on the inside of your left thigh. Bring your hands into prayer position at your heart centre, pressing your palms together and lifting your sternum to the thumbs, creating space for your baby and your internal organs.

Keep your gaze focused on one point and when you are stable, raise the arms up so your hands are parallel, palms facing. Lengthen the crown of the head, relax your shoulders and keep your standing leg strong. Here you become the tree of life – feel yourself strong and balanced, reaching to your highest potential and breathe well for 3–6 breaths.

When you are ready to come out, inhale and, as you exhale, place your palms together in prayer position above your head, then draw your hands down through your centre, and come back to your heart. Release your leg and take a few moments standing tall with one hand on your heart and one on your belly feeling truly blessed. Repeat on the other side.

MISCARRIAGE

A miscarriage is the loss of a baby before twenty-four weeks. It can be an extremely distressing experience and, sadly, early miscarriages (before twelve weeks) are very common. Some studies suggest that one in four pregnancies results in miscarriage. Often women don't even know they've miscarried, especially if they weren't trying for a baby or if they have an irregular cycle. Late miscarriages (after twelve weeks) are much rarer.

Nobody really knows what causes a miscarriage, but experts think that it's usually due to the baby not developing as it should or health issues with the mother, such as a problem with the placenta. The only lifestyle factors that will increase your risk are things like smoking, alcohol, excessive amounts of caffeine and illegal drugs.

Nearly all of you will know somebody who has had a miscarriage. While we were writing this book my wife Christiane suffered one. Here's her story.

CHRISTIANE'S STORY

'Charlotte was nine months old when we felt ready to try for another baby. I felt like my body was strong enough, I'd recovered from pregnancy and childbirth and I was finally getting some sleep. In July 2012 I missed a period and took a test right away which came back positive. Because we'd struggled for so long to conceive Charlotte, we were very excited and told our friends and family straight away. Knowing that Charlotte was soon going to have a little brother or sister to play with made me so happy. Because my pregnancy with her had been straightforward and because I'm a positive person, I just expected everything to be OK.

'I had a scan at around eight weeks and at first the doctor said the baby didn't look big enough. Then they told us the devastating news that they couldn't find a heartbeat. They thought it had happened at around seven weeks. A week later I had the most awful cramping and bleeding as I miscarried our baby. I was crushed, and looked for a reason. Was it that yoga class I took or all the travelling we'd been doing? I think women often look for a reason for these things and blame themselves, but my doctor reassured me it was "just one of those things". It's often just the body's way of not going through with an unhealthy pregnancy or baby.

'Luckily I had James's support, and having to get up each day and care for Charlotte helped enormously – looking after her helped take my mind off things and kept me busy. That's not to say I wasn't devastated. I so badly wanted another baby, not just for us, but for Charlotte too. And a close friend announced her pregnancy soon after and her due date was the same as mine would have been. That was incredibly tough. But I've tried to stay positive and I've told myself things happen in life for a reason. Sometimes that reason is hard to see, but it all becomes apparent in time. I trust in the universe and my body. And I know that little soul will come back to us again some day in another baby and I can't wait.'

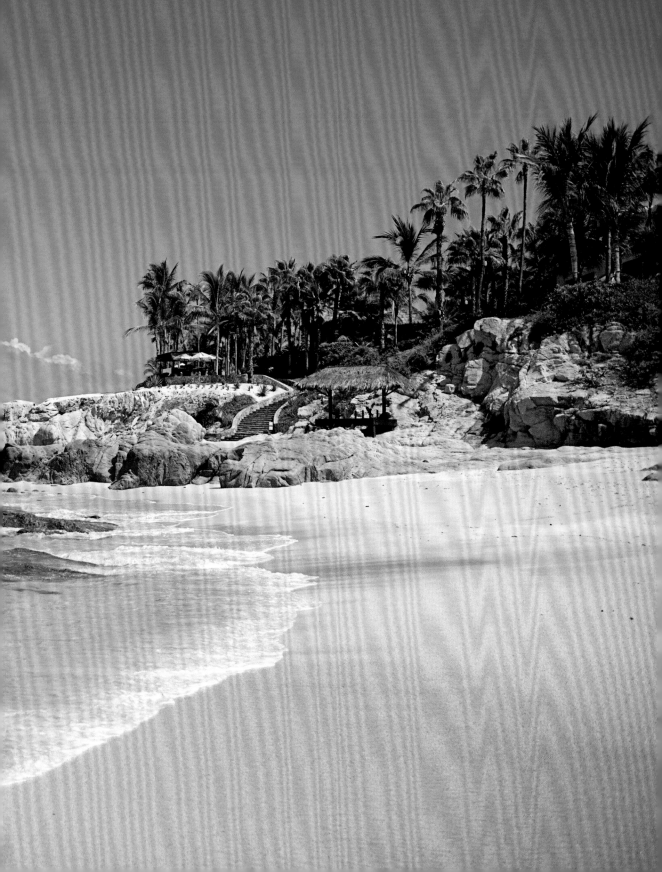

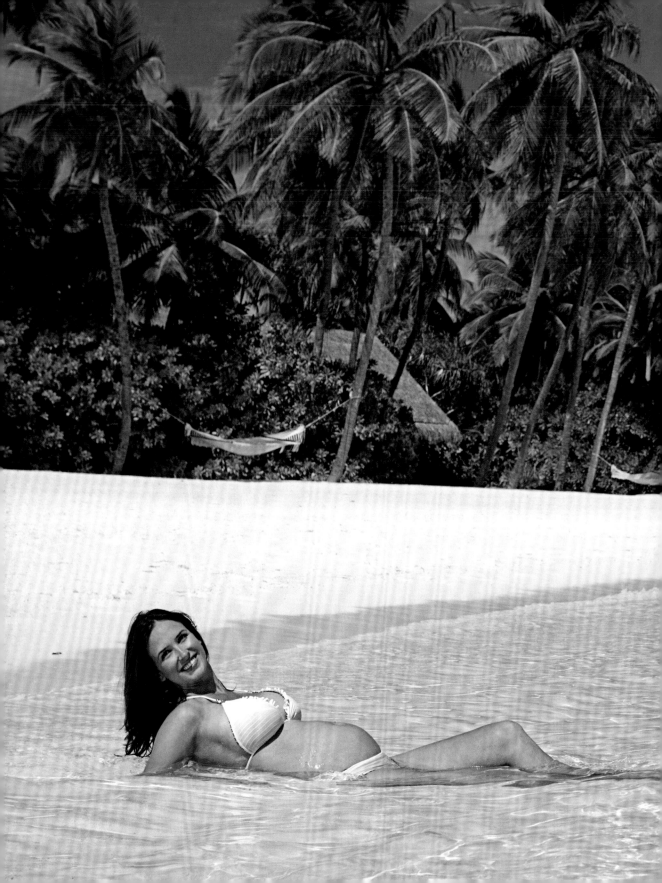

CHAPTER 4

THE SECOND TRIMESTER

WEEKS 13–28

The second trimester describes the period of pregnancy between weeks 13 and 28 and it's often the time when women say they feel their best. It's also when your bump starts to look like a bump, and you don't just look bloated and out of shape! The nausea, cravings and tiredness from the first twelve weeks (the first trimester) have usually eased up. And your bump isn't as heavy or uncomfortable as it might be in the third trimester, so the middle part of pregnancy is often the easiest. For this reason, now is the best time to include some safe exercise into your weekly routine and eat as healthily as possible.

The old saying, 'You're eating for two,' really isn't true, so continue to eat Clean & Lean throughout the second trimester. Of course, that's not to say you should diet – I'd never advocate that in pregnancy – but try not to binge on sugary snacks or junk food. It's all about being kind to yourself; in fact, you're being kind for two now. So nourish yourself and always choose what works best for you. Your body will thank you for it because eating a healthy, balanced diet now will help you sleep better, make you feel better and will be better for your baby. Plus, you won't have to lose all the extra weight when you have had your baby – when you will have neither the time nor the energy to lose the extra pounds. So don't eat lots of cake in the mistaken belief that you 'need it'. You don't. What you need are lots of vitamins, minerals and nourishing foods to keep you and baby healthy.

FROM THE MIDWIFE

'At the start of this trimester your baby is around 9cm long. If it's a girl, her ovarian follicles are beginning to form, and, if it's a boy, his prostate starts to appear. Your baby's body is developing a skeleton which begins to harden as the weeks go on. At around seventeen weeks, fat starts to accumulate under your baby's skin, which will provide him or her with energy and will eventually keep them warm after birth. In the second trimester they start to hear and their eyes start to move. At around nineteen weeks, vernix caseosa, a greasy whitish coating, begins to form all over your baby as a protection. Most of this is shed before they're born, but some babies are born with a little left on their skin. Towards the end of this trimester you may be able to feel your baby's movements – sooner if it's your second or third pregnancy. They'll start off feeling like flutters and get firmer as your baby grows bigger and stronger.'
BY JULIE SCHILLER

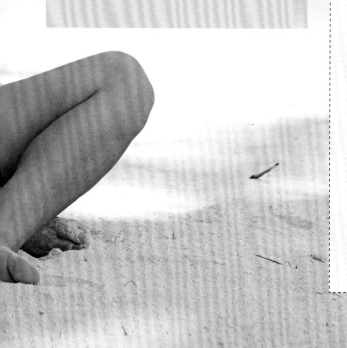

YOUR DIET IN THE SECOND TRIMESTER

As well as eating many of the usual Clean & Lean foods, there are some other things you should bear in mind during the second trimester. So let's start with a few tips:

✳ **Eat more chromium-rich foods:** The body needs this trace mineral to stabilise blood-sugar levels; insufficient chromium can lead to sugar cravings and tiredness. So try to eat chromium-rich foods, including sunflower seeds, quinoa, brown rice and oats.

✳ **Eat more magnesium:** According to research, many women are deficient in magnesium and feel stressed and anxious as a result. Some studies also suggest that morning sickness can be related to a lack of magnesium. It's found in the same foods as chromium.

✳ **Don't be fat phobic:** If you've previously had a low-fat diet, this needs to stop in pregnancy. You need plenty of foods containing good fats (e.g. avocados and nuts) and good oils (e.g. avocado, flaxseed and walnut oil), and make sure your pregnancy supplement contains omega-3 (most do).

✳ **Vitamin D:** Continue to take a 10 mcg supplement each day to help your baby develop strong bones.

BODY IMAGE

I know from my clients – and from Christiane – that pregnancy can throw up a lot of issues surrounding body image. On the one hand, you're thrilled to be having a baby, but on the other hand, putting on weight, thinking you are unattractive and feeling you're losing control of your body can be daunting. It doesn't make you vain or ungrateful – it's perfectly natural. So try to embrace your new curves, dress them well, stay healthy and treat yourself, if you can, to anything that makes you feel good – like a blow-dry, manicure or pregnancy massage. But not everyone has the time for or can afford a treat, so let me just say to you right now – you're amazing, what you are doing is amazing and you are my hero.

UNWANTED ADVICE

When you're pregnant, it can often feel like you have an invisible sign around your neck that says, 'Please give me advice! And don't forget to tell me all the gory details about your delivery!'

Everybody thinks they're an expert on pregnancy and raising children, but in reality, every pregnancy, birth and child are different, so just smile and thank them, then go ahead and do what feels right for you. Christiane and I politely avoided negativity and people who seemed to delight in telling frightening stories. Don't let people scare you with stories about their nine-day labour or what you should do once baby is here. The only expert out there for you and your baby is you.

*top tip

Start massaging oil into your breasts, bump, bottom and thighs every day. This will help to reduce the appearance of stretch marks and is a lovely way to bond with your bump.

'STAYING FIT HELPED ME PREPARE FOR LABOUR'

'As a model and performance specialist at Bodyism I've always aimed to live Clean & Lean. When I found out that I was pregnant it felt great to know that the Clean & Lean lifestyle was going to make me feel energised and healthy during the pregnancy, and it was also reassuring to know that my baby boy was getting the best possible start in my tummy.

'I changed my diet and exercise programme slightly during my pregnancy. For example, I introduced a few more healthy carbohydrates to my meals and I stopped drinking coffee completely for the first six months. I did pregnancy yoga twice a week and performed a Bodyism pregnancy exercise routine three times a week. I also walked to work most days, which took me around 30 minutes.

'I tried to have a massage or reflexology once a week to prevent any aches and to calm my system down. It was a great combination for me to stay healthy and flexible during the pregnancy and it also gave me breathing techniques that helped during labour.

'It's difficult to imagine what a pregnant woman is going through until you've been there yourself. Now I've experienced a pregnancy it feels even easier to help my pregnant clients at Bodyism. With the help of this book, you too can feel amazing during and post pregnancy and create a happy and healthy baby! Good luck with your pregnancy!'
by Nathalie Schyllert, director of operations and senior performance specialist at Bodyism

EXERCISE IN THE SECOND TRIMESTER

EXERCISE TIPS

During your second trimester, avoid lying on your back, either during exercise or when you're sleeping as the weight of your uterus presses on the major vein that returns blood from your lower body to your heart. This can make you feel dizzy and could interfere with the flow of blood and nutrients to the placenta and your developing baby.

Perform the workout below three times a week on non-consecutive days. On days between your workouts, go for a brisk walk or a light swim. Your workouts should last no longer than 30–45 minutes, and you must be sure to listen to your body and take plenty of rest between sets. Relax, enjoy and be kind to yourself and the little bundle of love you are carrying. You're a superhero, but even superheroes need to take it easy.

Note: See pages 62–3 for advice on exercise during pregnancy and seek guidance from your GP or health professional if you are in any doubt about exercising.

EXERCISE	REPS	SETS	REST
Superman	10–15/side	1	30–60 secs
Side-lying single-leg knee-raise with mini-band	10–15/side	1	30–60 secs
Mini-band walking	10–15/side	1	30–60 secs
Y	10–15	1	30–60 secs
T	12–15	2–3	30–60 secs
Goddess squat	8–10	2–3	30–60 secs
Arm extension with mini-band	12–15	2–3	30–60 secs
Arm circle	12–15	2–3	30–60 secs

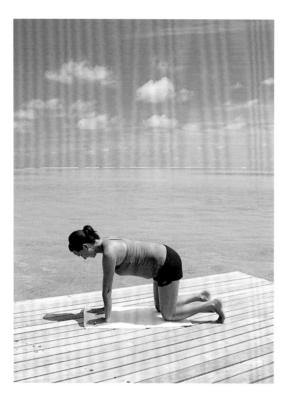
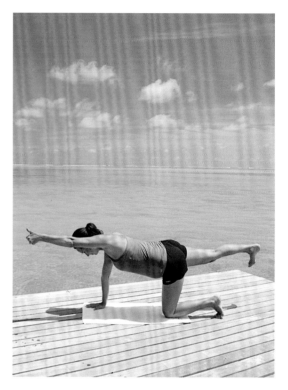

Superman

Start position: Support yourself on your hands and knees with hands under shoulders and knees under hips and with your toes firmly pointed into the floor. Ensure your spine and neck are in a straight line by keeping your gaze to the floor, just in front of your fingertips.

The movement: Extend your left arm out in front of you beyond your head, thumb up, while extending your right leg backwards – imagine you are being pulled from either end. Return to the start position and repeat 10–15 times on each side.

*top tip

To keep your lower back safe, imagine trying to lengthen your arm and leg out in a line away from your body whilst keeping your hips parallel to the floor.

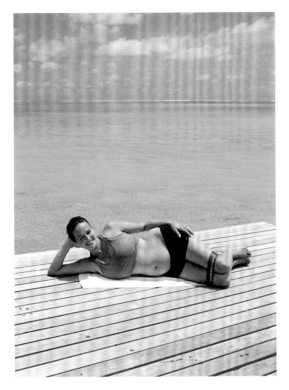

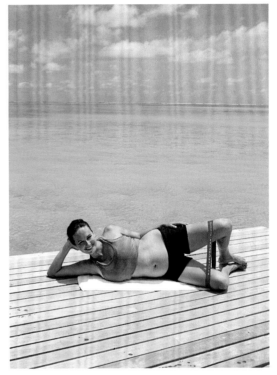

Side-lying single-leg knee-raise with mini-band

Start position: Place a Bodyism mini-band around both legs just above your knees. Lie on your right side, bend your right elbow and rest your head on your right hand. Bend your knees to a 90-degree angle and stack them on top of one another. Keep your body in line and engage your core by pulling your belly button in towards your spine.

The movement: Raise your top knee by pushing against the resistance of the mini-band. Take the knee up as far as you can without straining the lower back, keeping both feet together. With control, slowly lower back to the start position. Repeat 10–15 times on each side.

*top tip

This strengthens your butt muscles, which need to be strong to help keep your lower back supported and healthy as the size of your bump increases.

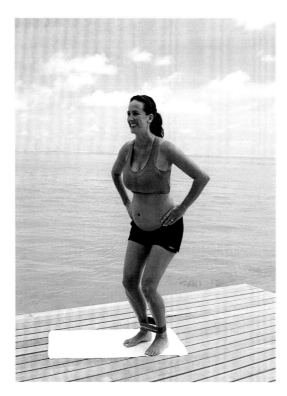
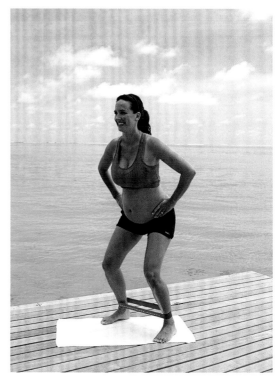

Mini-band walking

Start position: Take a Bodyism mini-band of your chosen strength and place it just above your ankles. Stand with your feet hip-width apart, hands resting on your hips, and engage the core by pulling your belly button in towards your spine.

The movement: Take one large step out sideways to the right, keeping the legs straight and without using your body for momentum. Then bring your left foot in half a step, keeping tension in the band all the time. Repeat this movement for 10 steps on each side.

*top tip
This exercise helps reduce the risk of knee pain, which can affect you as your bump begins to grow.

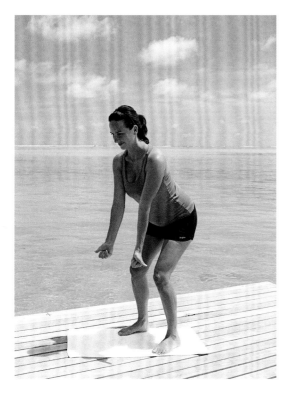 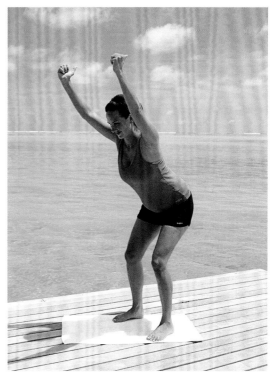

Y

Start position: Stand with your feet hip-width apart, bend your knees and stick your bottom out, so your upper body leans forwards 45 degrees. Hold your hands directly below your chest with fists clenched and thumbs up, keeping your head and back in a straight line, your shoulders back and down. Engage your core by pulling your belly button in towards the spine.

The movement: Raise both hands to create a 'Y' shape above your head with your arms by your ears, then return to the starting point. Repeat 10–15 times.

*top tip
This exercise targets the muscles between the shoulder blades that need to be strong for when you have a baby to hold.

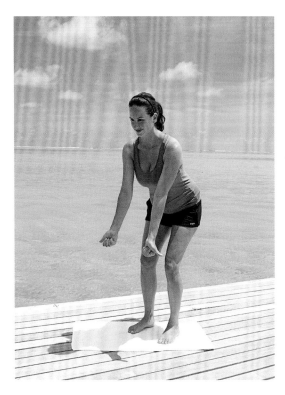
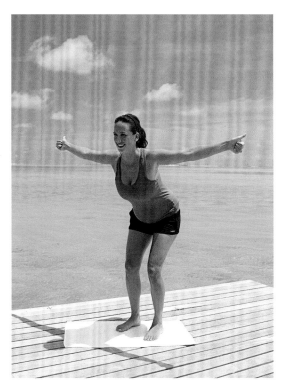

T

Start position: Stand with your feet hip-width apart.
Bend your knees and lean forwards so your torso is
at a 45 degree angle. Keep your head and back in a
straight line, your shoulders back and down and your
hands directly below your chest with fists clenched and
thumbs pointing outwards. Engage your core by pulling
your belly button in towards the spine.

The movement: Keeping your body still and your core
engaged, raise your arms out to the side to form a 'T'
shape, then return to the start position. Repeat 8–10 times.

*top tip
This exercise will strengthen your
upper back – perfect if you have
found your posture deteriorating.
Ensure you maintain a flat back
throughout the movement.

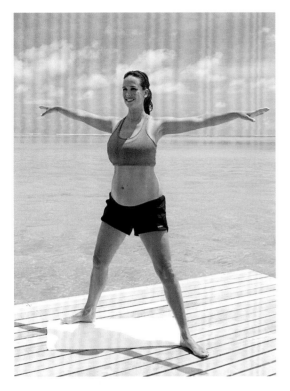 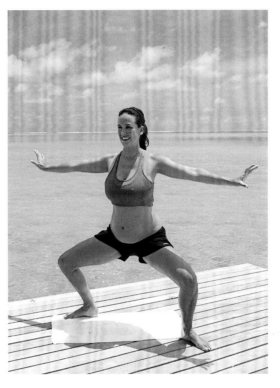

Goddess squat

Start position: Take a comfortable stance with your feet slightly wider than shoulder-width apart, toes pointing outward, core engaged (by pulling your belly button in towards your spine). Raise your arms to the side, level with your shoulders and palms facing down.

The movement: Inhale and bend your knees directly over your toes and lower your hips into a squat, aiming to bring your thighs parallel to the floor. Keep your arms extended out to the sides at shoulder height, with palms facing down. Keep your chest open and hips pushed back. Exhale as you push through your heels to return to the start position. Repeat 8–10 times.

*top tip

Women who do squats may have an easier time during labour due to the similarities in movement between squatting and giving birth.

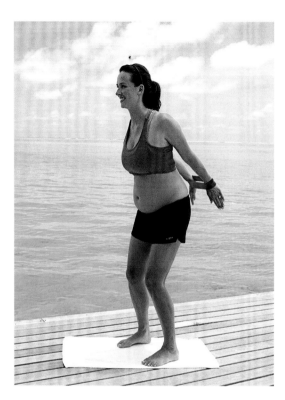

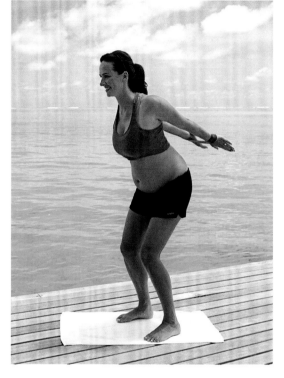

Arm extension with mini-band

Start position: Place a Bodyism mini-band around both of your wrists and take your arms out behind your back. Standing, take a comfortable stance with your feet shoulder-width apart and your knees bent, then hinge forward slightly at your hips. Engage the core by pulling your belly button in towards the spine.

The movement: Push against the resistance of the mini-band, taking your arms up as far away from your body as you can and return to the start position. Repeat 12–15 times.

*top tip
This exercise is great for strengthening your shoulders, arms and upper back.

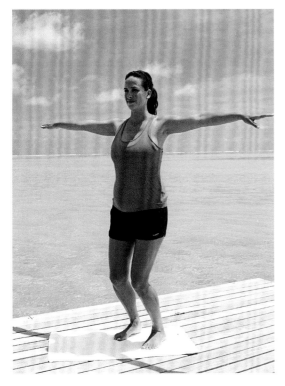 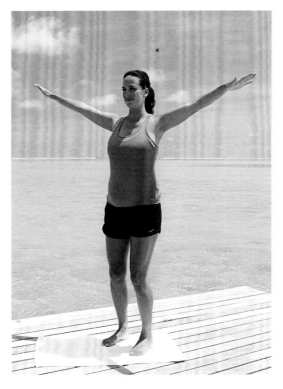

Arm circle

Start position: Stand with your feet shoulder-width apart and knees slightly bent. Hold your arms out at shoulder height, parallel to the floor, and keep your core engaged by pulling your belly button in towards your spine.

The movement: Keeping the movement small, circle the arms forward 12–15 times, then repeat in the opposite direction, without taking a break if you can.

*top tip

This will help increase the endurance in your shoulder muscles, which in turn will make it easier to hold your baby for longer. Be sure not to hunch your upper back or use your torso for momentum.

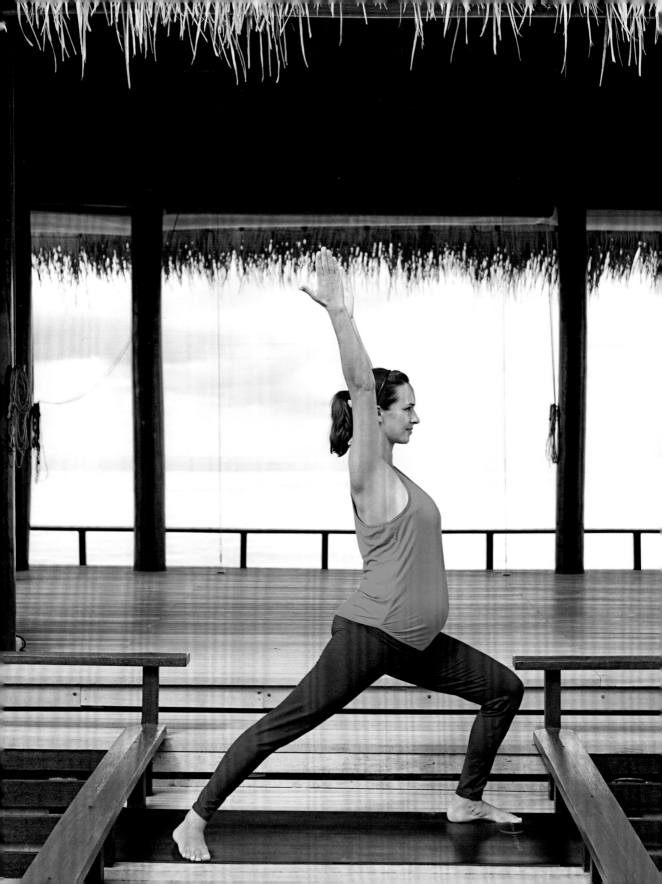

YOGA IN THE SECOND TRIMESTER

BY WENCHE BEARD

'The second trimester of your pregnancy may be your favourite part. Your energy levels will probably rise again and you'll start to "look" pregnant. You'll also begin to feel your baby for the first time! For this part of your pregnancy I have chosen some standing postures for strength and stability, bringing about a feeling of empowerment.'

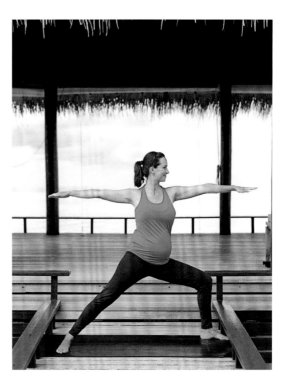

Virabhadrasana I (Peaceful warrior pose I)

Begin standing tall, feet together. Take a moment to acknowledge what it feels like to stand tall and breathe well. Turn your right foot outward to a 45-degree angle and step forward with your left leg, hips level to the front. Keep your hands on your hips and inhale. Then, as you exhale, bend your right knee, keeping it over the ankle.

Drop your arms by the side of your body and relax your shoulders. Inhale and let the arms rise along the ears, palms facing each other; keep your fingers alive.

If you want to take it into a gentle back bend, create space from the soles of your feet to the fingertips as you inhale and, as you exhale, gently lift your face and heart to the sky as you keep your shoulders melting down your back. Stay with an open heart for 3–6 breaths, celebrating the gift of your pregnancy. Come back on an inhale, exhale and lower your arms. Step together and sway your hips to relieve the back before repeating the posture on the other side.

Virabhadrasana II (Warrior pose II)

Begin standing tall, feet together. Walk your feet wide, with your hands on your hips. Turn your left foot out 90 degrees, making sure your left heel is in line with your right instep and your hips are level to the front.

Inhale and, as you exhale, bend the left knee over the left ankle. Drop your arms by the side of your body and, on the inhale, raise your arms parallel to the floor, extending from your collar bones, through the armpits to the fingertips.

Relax your shoulders down your back, legs rotating outward as you gather energy up to your pelvis, lifting your baby and keeping the legs strong as you gaze down your left fingertips. Breathe well here for 3–6 breaths as you let the strength of your body empower you. Feel the energy of endurance as you prepare for the birth of your baby. Be mindful of your balance here. Inhale as you come out of the posture and, as you exhale, lower your arms before you slowly come back to standing tall. Stay here for a few breaths before you repeat on the other side.

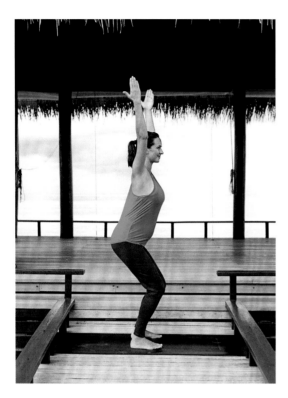

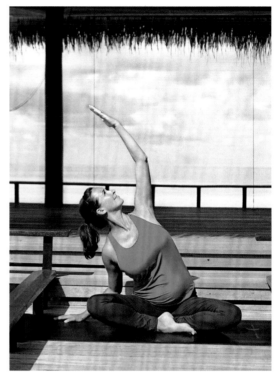

Utkatasana (Chair pose)

Stand tall with your feet firmly grounded, crown of your head to the sky and feel your baby at the very centre of your body. Inhale as you let the arms rise to the sky, palms facing, fingers alive, shoulders relaxed.

Exhale as you bend your knees and begin to sit back as if you were sitting onto a chair. Anchor your tailbone down towards your heels and hug your baby to your spine so you don't overarch your lower back. Keep the sides of your body long and feel space through your spine to the tips of your fingers. Enjoy a spacious body, rising from the strong foundation of your legs. Stay for 3–6 breaths.

On an inhale, slowly straighten the legs and, as you exhale, lower the arms and return to standing tall, breathing a breath that is supporting your strength and your baby's strength. If there is tension in the shoulders, keep your hands on your hips or rest them on your thighs.

Sukhasana side stretch (Easy pose side stretch)

Sit cross-legged (or with your legs wide if you prefer) with your arms by your side.

Practise a long spine and bring your right hand on to the floor. As you inhale, let the left hand rise to the sky along the left side of the body.

As you exhale, slowly lean over to the right side and lift and rotate your upper chest, gazing upwards at the sky. Stay for 3–6 breaths, breathing into the left side of your body. Come back to the centre on an inhale and repeat on the other side.

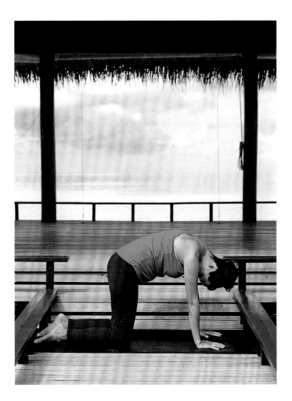

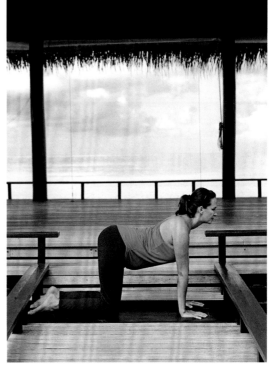

Marjaryasana/Bitilasana (Cat pose/Cow pose)

Start in a 'table-top' position with your palms under your shoulders and your knees directly under your hips. Look down to the floor, keeping your neck long.

Breathe in to a long spine and, as you exhale, begin to turn your tailbone down towards the floor as you round your spine towards the sky and hug your baby to the spine, gathering energy through your pelvis. Keep space between your shoulder blades and relax your head.

Inhale and turn your tailbone to the sky as you begin to arch the spine, letting your baby relax in the hammock of your belly as you move your heart forward, inviting the breath all the way to your baby.

You can continue this very soothing flow back and forth for as long as you feel comfortable, soothing out any tension in the back. When you decide to finish, sit back on to your heels with your legs apart, resting with your head on the floor and relaxed arms.

*top tip

This is a wonderful pose to return to again and again, even in labour with some lovely tail wagging.

CHAPTER 5

THE THIRD TRIMESTER

WEEKS 29–40

*top tip

This may sound obvious, but I'm going to say it anyway – pack your hospital bag early this trimester. Unless you're planning a home birth, in which case just get everything you need in place.

FROM THE MIDWIFE

'At the start of this trimester, your baby is around 25cm long and weighs just over 2lb. Your baby may have hair at this point and their bones are fully formed but still soft. At 32 weeks your baby's toe and finger nails have developed. The soft, downy hair – lanugo – that has been covering your baby will start to fall out at this point and their skin will become less wrinkled as more fat begins to form. Babies rapidly gain weight in the last few weeks of pregnancy. By 38 weeks your baby is considered full-term and could be born at any time. The lungs will continue to develop until birth and the baby will probably weigh between 6 and 10lb in the last few weeks.'

BY JULIE SCHILLER

YOUR DIET IN THE THIRD TRIMESTER

During the last trimester you'll need around 450 extra calories a day (this is just an approximate guide and varies depending on whether you were over- or underweight before you got pregnant – if in doubt, speak to your doctor). As ever, it's best to obtain the extra calories from the most nutritious foods you can find, so you and baby get plenty of lovely vitamins and minerals, rather than using pregnancy as an excuse to eat lots of cake. But my advice is to not get too hung up on calories and instead just listen to your body, eating when you feel hungry and choosing from a wide range of Clean & Lean foods.

Snacking is especially important around now; you may find yourself becoming increasingly tired, and regular small meals will help keep your blood-sugar levels steady and your energy levels up. Your growing baby is also putting pressure on your stomach, so you may find large meals make you feel uncomfortable, bloated, gassy and cause heartburn (sounds like a lot of men I know – surely they're not all pregnant!). So eat little and often.

Official advice says that women who were a healthy weight pre-pregnancy should aim to gain between 25 and 35lb throughout the whole of their pregnancy. Underweight women should aim for 28 to 40lb, and overweight women 15 to 25lb – slightly less if they were obese before becoming pregnant. Having said that, when my clients ask me about weight gain in pregnancy, my advice is always the same – don't worry about the scales, just focus on eating a healthy, balanced diet and keep in mind that you are doing something beautiful and amazing.

In my experience, women tend to gain weight differently during their pregnancies. Some gain only baby weight, while others lay down a lot of fat on their hips or other areas; some hold on to a lot of fluid and can suffer from bloating, while others find their breasts become very large, which can show up on the scales. Some women are genetically predisposed to have larger babies, others have smaller babies. Every woman and every pregnancy is different, so it's important not to compare yourself to other pregnant women. Just focus on good health, for yourself and your baby, and everything else will take care of itself.

*top tip

Take your rings off towards the end of your pregnancy – especially precious ones like your engagement ring, if you have one. Fluid retention may cause fingers to swell and rings to become stuck. If you end up having to have a C-section they'll ask you to remove jewellery and if you can't remove your rings yourself they may have to be cut off. So take them off around now and store them somewhere safe.

FIVE ENERGY-BOOSTING STAPLES

✳ **Eggs** – the yolks are a rich source of B vitamins, which convert food into energy. They're also a fantastic source of protein which helps keep you full (hunger can cause dips in energy). Remember, however, to cook them well – avoid runny yolks so have your eggs hard-boiled, well scrambled or in an omelette.

✳ **Nuts** – the healthy fat they contain provides a good source of long-lasting energy. Good fats also keep you full, so always keep your favourite nuts handy to snack on.

✳ **Water** – one of the leading but most overlooked causes of tiredness is dehydration. In pregnancy it's important to stay hydrated because water helps deliver nutrients from your food to your growing baby. So drink plenty of still, filtered water every day. Have it warm in the morning (with a slice of lemon) to flush out your system and help ward off any common pregnancy complaints like constipation, or with lemon or cucumber slices during the day.

✳ **Quinoa** – this is incredibly high in protein as well as being a complex carbohydrate, so it provides you with long-lasting energy throughout the day. You can add it to soups, casseroles, risottos and salads and even make a muesli from it, adding berries.

✳ **Pumpkin seeds** – these are a fantastic source of magnesium and zinc which helps increase energy levels. Snack on them or sprinkle them over your food.

FIVE ENERGY-DRAINERS

✳ **Biscuits/cookies** – don't fall into the trap of perking yourself up after a tiring day with a biscuit. Foods high in sugar might give you an instant hit of energy by quickly raising your blood-sugar levels, but these effects are fleeting, and when your blood-sugar levels crash you'll feel even more tired than before.

✳ **Salty foods** – too much salt dehydrates you, which causes tiredness, so avoid crisps, salted peanuts, processed foods and ready meals. The last two in particular are often packed with hidden salt.

✳ **Breakfast cereals** – if you've read my previous Clean & Lean books, or the introduction to Clean & Lean in Chapter 1, you'll know that I'm not a fan of most commercial breakfast cereals. They're marketed as an energising start to your day, but in reality they're lacking in nutrients and packed with sugar. A plain porridge mixed with chopped nuts and berries is a far healthier – and more energising – option for breakfast.

✳ **Fizzy drinks** – these are incredibly high in sugar, so, like biscuits and cookies, they might give you a fleeting burst of energy, but they will leave you even more tired. Recent studies have also suggested that some of them can lower your mood because of the artificial sweeteners they contain. Many also contain caffeine, which you should limit in pregnancy.

✳ **Fried food** – studies show that fatty, fried foods like takeaway chips and burgers cause fatigue, increased grogginess and daytime sleepiness. And that's the last thing you need in your final trimester!

*top tip

Fill your home with healthy snacks for now and the first weeks of motherhood. Make sure you have plenty of fruit, nuts, seeds, oatcakes and vegetables – and ask visitors to bring them too.

HOLLY VALANCE

'So I'm 36 weeks preggers and not only am I taken over by a mutant alien, I'm supposed to do it with a huge grateful smile on my dial. And quite frankly... it's petrifying. My body now belongs to a very demanding blob who's been on my wish list for some time, yes, BUT also makes my nose bleed daily, nod off at dinner, forget what you told me 3 minutes ago and walk around like an old lady with nasty pelvic pains – and that's just the first 12 weeks. Ha!

'The movies only mention the nausea, cravings and cankles. No one mentions the leaky boobs, bad skin, crying randomly at nappy ads, the murderous thoughts when looking at ones' partner (*Gawd, no one would dare – we'd never do it!*). But you know what? We do, and thankfully the glorious "baby brain", making me as thick as two planks, will make sure I want another one after this too!

'I worry weekly, "Am I putting on enough weight? Am I putting on too much??" I'm lucky that my cravings have mainly been healthy – veggie juices and Vegemite toast, but I admit that chocolate fills a void in my life regularly and don't ever argue with a pregnant lady if she needs ice-cream! There are so many conflicting and often strict ideas out there on what to eat/wear/consume/attempt while pregnant that your head is just bombarded with way too many concepts that work wonderfully for some, but awfully for you.

'Therefore, be open to guidance and then do what feels best for you. You're going to read this book and have great days that make you feel wonderful, like you're conquering the world. Then the next day may be off-kilter, but you MUST keep going on your path, because you want this, it's why you picked this book up to begin with, and you can keep making good choices, most of the time! Your baby only needs "healthy Mummy", not "svelte Mummy", and she will come naturally with a little patience and practicality. Your mind needs to be thinking clearly and calmly – not pressured with guilt that you might not be doing it right.

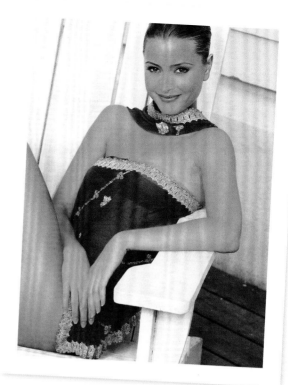

'What's right anyway? Seven billion of us got here didn't we, and the chances are that noone in a yurt in remote Mongolia reads the pregnancy guidelines on avoiding sushi, nail polish and tummy sleeping. And they do alright. There ISN'T one way, there are just "ways". You'll find *yours*.'

UPDATE: 'So, my little girl Luka is now 3 months old and, well.... they were right. It was ALL worth it. Every last ache and whingey pain. All the things that I used to panic and worry about have gone poof, out of the window. WHO. CARES? There's a new No. 1 in town! I'm now very focused on an extremely important little person who is a brilliant incentive to look after my body and mind so I can be a great Mummy. If I want to create a kind, thoughtful and loving human, I have to be all those things to myself too. I need to nourish my body as well as I can most days, and if I falter, be kind enough to let it go and keep trying my best...it's all any of us can do.

XXX'

WORKING OUT IN THE THIRD TRIMESTER

If you feel up to it, carry on exercising during your last trimester, although – as with the rest of your pregnancy – you must listen to your body and continue only if you feel up to it. If you feel tired, choose sleep over exercise. And stay in touch with a health professional you trust – speak to your midwife, doula or doctor at any time if you have any concerns in your last trimester.

The exercises I've chosen for you to try during the third trimester avoid any lying on your back, and can also help prevent symphysis pubis dysfunction (SPD). The symphysis pubis is the joint that connects your pelvis joints; during pregnancy your body produces more of a hormone called relaxin which softens the ligaments that hold together and strengthen your pelvis (to prepare it for childbirth) and a gap in the pubic joint can widen too far, causing inflammation and pain.

The workouts in your third trimester are all about you moving in a safe way that doesn't lead to overexertion. The exercises in the workout below switch on the important postural muscles. Perform them three times a week on non-consecutive days for no longer than 30 minutes. On the days in between your workouts, go for a brisk walk or a light swim.

*top tip
As always, listen to your body and take plenty of rest between sets.

EXERCISE	REPS	SETS	REST
Superman	10–15/side	1	30–60 secs
Side-lying single-leg knee-raise with mini-band	10–15/side	1	30–60 secs
Y	10–15	1	30–60 secs
T	12–15	1–2	30–60 secs
Energy push	8–10	1–2	30–60 secs
Arm circle	12–15	2–3	30–60 secs

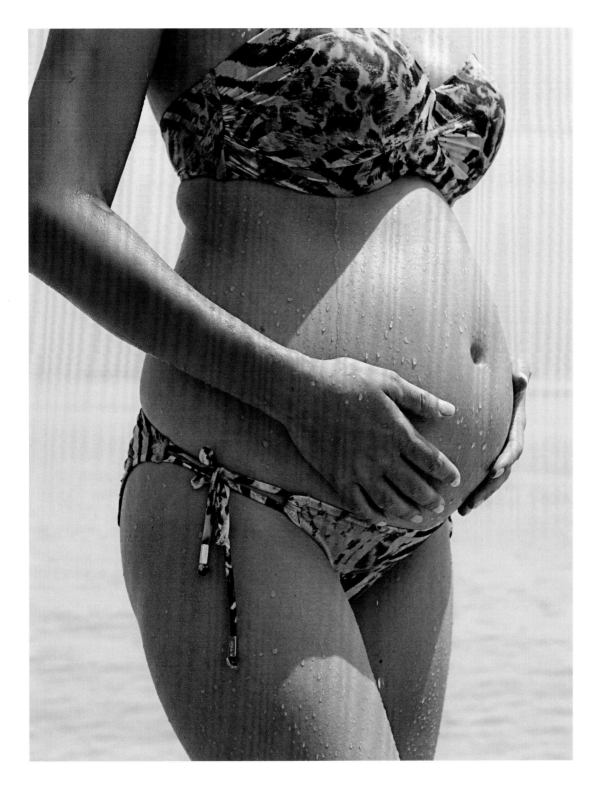

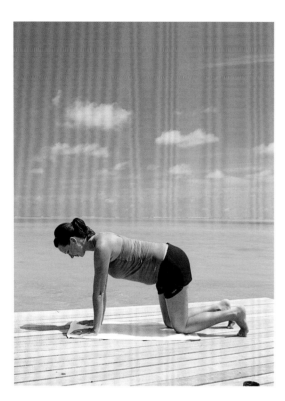
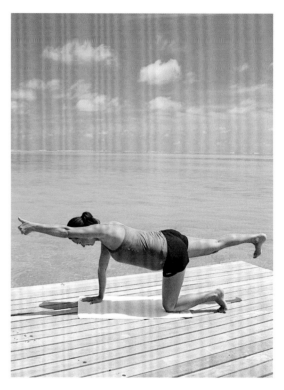

Superman

Start position: Support yourself on your hands and knees with hands under shoulders and knees under hips and with your toes firmly pointed into the floor. Ensure your spine and neck are in a straight line by keeping your gaze to the floor, just in front of your fingertips.

The movement: Extend your left arm out in front of you beyond your head, thumb up, while extending your right leg backwards – imagine you are being pulled from either end. Return to the start position and repeat 10–15 times on each side.

*top tip

This exercise will activate and strengthen your hamstrings, glutes and lower-back muscles, as well as improve your overall body balance.

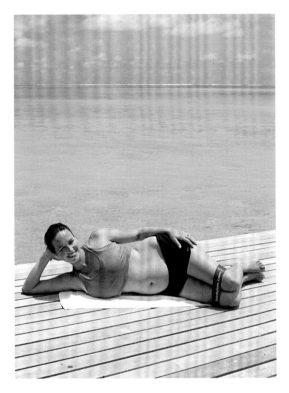 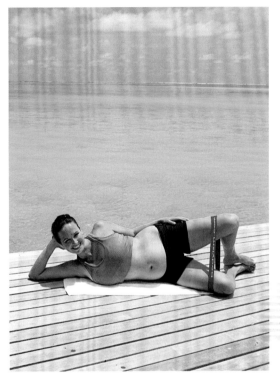

Side-lying single-leg knee-raise with mini-band

Start position: Place a Bodyism mini-band around both legs just above your knees. Lie on your right side, bend your elbow and rest your head on your right hand. Bend your knees to a 90-degree angle and stack them on top of one another. Keep your body in line and engage your core by pulling your belly button in towards your spine.

The movement: Raise your top knee by pushing against the resistance of the mini-band. Take the knee up as far as you can without straining the lower back, keeping both feet together. With control, slowly lower back to the start position. Repeat 10-15 times on each side.

*top tip

To make this exercise harder, slow down the movement and really squeeze the muscles.

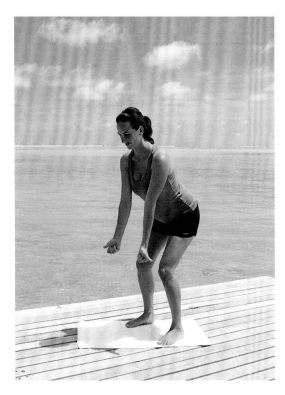
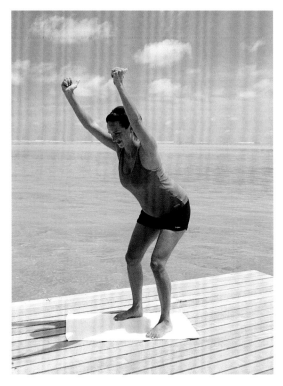

Y

Start position: Stand with your feet hip-width apart, bend your knees and stick your bottom out, so your upper body leans forwards 45 degrees. Hold your hands directly below your chest with fists clenched and thumbs up, keeping your head and back in a straight line, your shoulders back and down. Engage your core by pulling your belly button in towards the spine.

The movement: Raise both hands to create a 'Y' shape above your head with your arms by your ears, then return to the starting point. Repeat 10–15 times.

*top tip

Go for a walk every day – if you feel up to it, of course. This is a great way of keeping fit and boosting your energy levels. Plus, the gravity will help your baby get into the right position for labour. In fact, pacing around during the early stages of labour can help speed things along, as your baby jiggles down into the right position and puts pressure on your cervix which helps it to dilate.

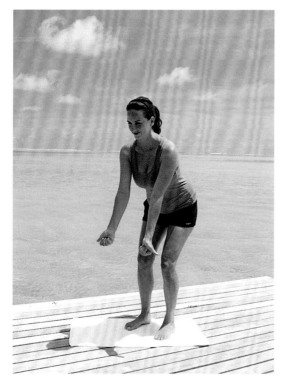
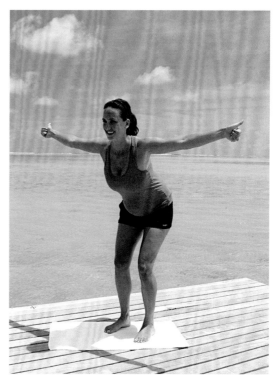

T

Start position: Stand with your feet hip-width apart. Bend your knees and lean forwards so your torso is at a 45-degree angle. Keep your head and back in a straight line, your shoulders back and down and your hands directly below your chest with fists clenched and thumbs pointing outward. Engage your core by pulling your belly button in towards the spine.

The movement: Keeping your body still and your core engaged, raise your arms out to the side to form a 'T' shape, then return to the start position. Repeat 12–15 times.

*top tip

This exercise will strengthen your upper back – perfect if you have found your posture deteriorating.

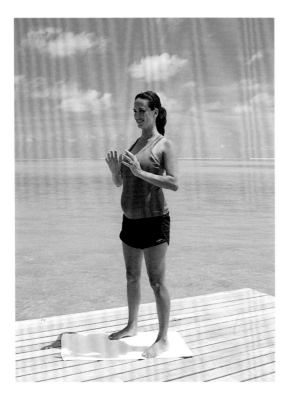
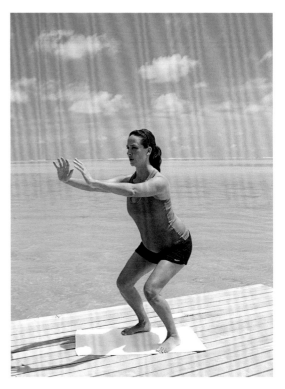

Energy push

Start position: Stand with your feet shoulder-width apart and your hands raised in front of your chest. Engage your core by pulling your belly button in towards the spine.

The movement: Exhale, bend the knees and push the hips back as you lower into a squat position. To stand up, push through the heels and bring the hips forwards as you inhale and bring your hands back in towards your body. Focus on breathing slowly and repeat 8–10 times.

*top tip
This exercise helps to improve digestion and is a natural energiser.

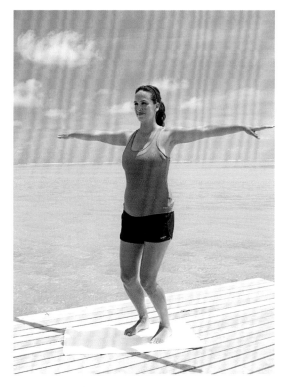

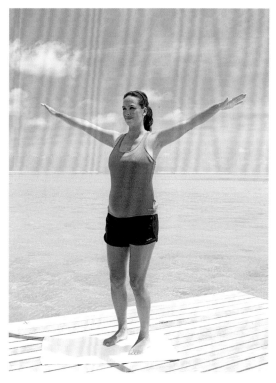

Arm circle

Start position: Stand with your feet shoulder-width apart and knees slightly bent. Hold your arms out at shoulder height, parallel to the floor, and keep your core engaged by pulling your belly button in towards your spine.

The movement: Keeping the movement small, circle the arms forward 12–15 times, then repeat in the opposite direction, without taking a break if you can.

*top tip

Exercising throughout your pregnancy has been shown to help reduce the risk of postpartum depression.

YOGA IN THE THIRD TRIMESTER

BY WENCHE BEARD

'By now your baby has grown considerably and is developing well. He or she is now "finalising" development, all snug in your "womb world", and you are moving more slowly. Give yourself permission to ease up as you enter the last part of your pregnancy, avoiding any postures that compress your belly. I have chosen postures that can be helpful in late pregnancy. As ever, do these exercises only if you feel up to it.

'This yoga programme has been developed so you can safely practise all of the postures throughout your pregnancy. Use props such as blocks, pillows and blankets as needed, making your practice as delightful as possible.

'Always listen to your body. Women who practise yoga during pregnancy are often more comfortable in their body, knowing how to relax and turn their awareness into their inner landscape, listening to their own body's natural rhythm, which really helps in labour. The more relaxed you are, the easier the descent of your baby moving through your birth canal. Through the support of your breath and your connection from the inside of your body – feeling, not thinking – you will know how to make the decisions of when to push and when to hold to gather strength for your next contraction. Let your breath support the arrival of your little miracle as you meet him or her for the first time. Your body knows how to give birth – trust it and go with it. Send love and encouragement to your baby, letting your body, rather than the thinking mind, birth your baby. When you practise your yoga in pregnancy, you practise yoga with your baby at the very centre of your body.'

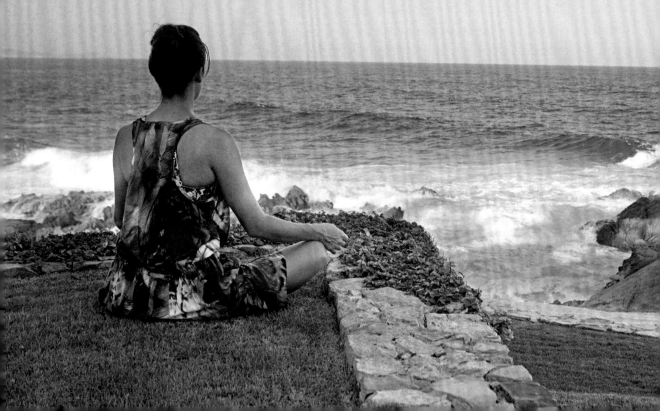

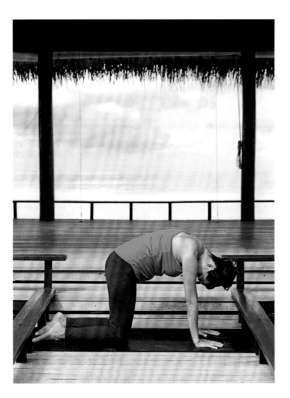

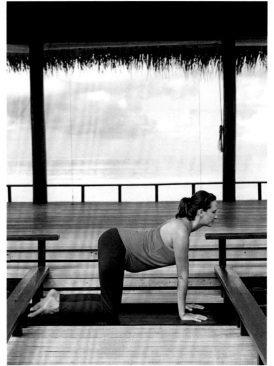

Marjaryasana/Bitilasana (Cat pose/Cow pose)

Start in a 'table-top' position with your palms under your shoulders and your knees directly under your hips. Look down to the floor, keeping your neck long.

Breathe in to a long spine and, as you exhale, begin to turn your tailbone down towards the floor as you round your spine towards the sky and hug your baby to the spine, gathering energy through your pelvis. Keep space between your shoulder blades and relax your head.

Inhale and turn your tailbone to the sky as you begin to arch the spine, letting your baby relax in the hammock of your belly as you move your heart forwards, inviting the breath all the way to your baby.

You can continue this very soothing flow back and forth for as long as you feel comfortable, soothing out any tension in the back. When you decide to finish, sit back on to your heels with your legs apart, resting with your head on the floor and relaxed arms.

*top tip
Don't forget, this is a wonderful pose to return to again and again, even in labour, with some lovely tail wagging.

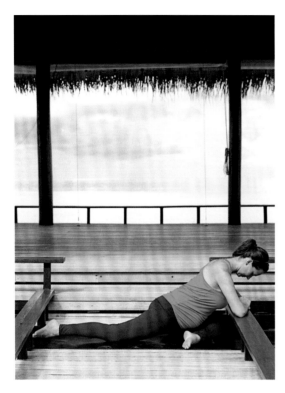

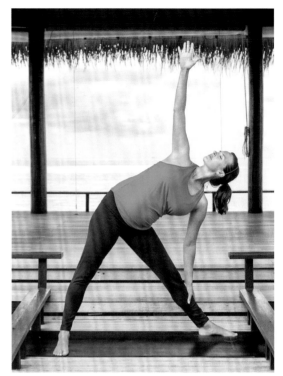

Eka pada rajakapotasana (Pigeon pose)

From 'table-top' position again, keep your hands beneath your shoulders and knees beneath your hips. Then bring your left leg forward with your knee towards your left hand and your left foot towards your right hip, making sure your baby has plenty of space. Use blocks, pillows or blankets for support to balance your hips out. Keep your right leg long behind you and your hands on the floor, supporting a long spine, broadening through your chest, with the back of your neck long and shoulders melting down that strong back.

Stay here for 3–6 breaths, opening through your hips, breathing into any tight spots and preparing for the birth of your baby. Come back by pushing on to your hands and, slowly, as you inhale, draw your left leg back and extend the foot behind you to stretch it out before moving to the other side.

Trikonasana (Triangle pose)

Stand tall, aware of your baby at the very centre of your body, then walk your feet about a metre or so apart, place your hands on your hips and turn your right foot 90 degrees, aligning your right heel with your left instep, hips level to the front.

Drop your arms by the side of your body and, as you inhale, lift the arms out to the side, parallel to the floor. As you exhale, draw back through the left hip as you extend your torso over your left leg with an open waist. Support yourself on your leg, blocks or even a chair if you need to. Reach up to the sky with your right arm, keeping your neck long and remembering your head is an extension of the spine.

Lengthen the tailbone towards your right heel, keep the legs strong, the spine long and arms active. Stay for 3–6 breaths, then come back on an inhale and lower the arms on the exhale. Take a few breaths here with your hands on your belly, embodying the state of balance for both you and your baby. Repeat the other side.

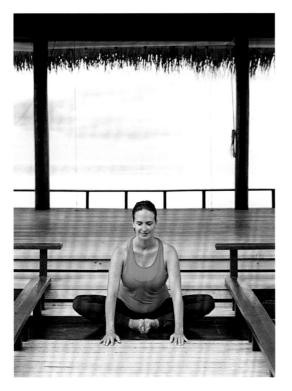

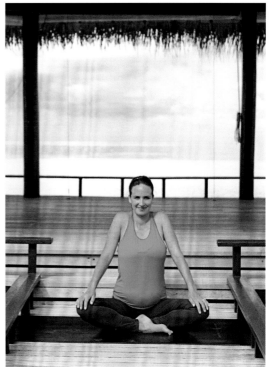

Buddha konasana (Bound-angle pose)

Begin by sitting on the floor, bending your knees and bringing the soles of your feet together with your heels towards your pelvis. Drop your knees out to the side, your pelvis spilling open, your spine rising from the earth to the sky. Close your eyes and breathe well.

From here you can come forwards into a forward bend to open your back as you curl over your baby, turning your awareness inward, opening your inner eye and looking down to your baby, spending some time with him or her. Stay for as long as is comfortable.

When you are ready to come out of the posture, return on an inhale and ground deep into the inner soil of your body as you exhale. Sit for a while before opening your eyes and bringing your legs together.

Neck and shoulder rolls – sitting or standing

Sit (or stand) in a comfortable position. If sitting, relax your hands on your knees and, if standing, relax your arms by your side. Feel the length of the spine and relax the shoulders. Inhale through the length of your spine and, as you exhale, drop the chin to the chest, gazing down to your baby. Stay here for a few breaths and with every exhale feel new space in the spine and neck.

Inhale as you let your head roll to your right shoulder, exhale as it falls back to the chest, then inhale as your head rolls to your left shoulder and exhale as it falls back to your chest. Let your head float from side to side with lightness and ease like a pendulum feeling the marriage of breath and movement for about 6 breaths.

Bring your head back to the centre and sit for a few moments, enjoying your peaceful body housing your miracle of love growing inside you.

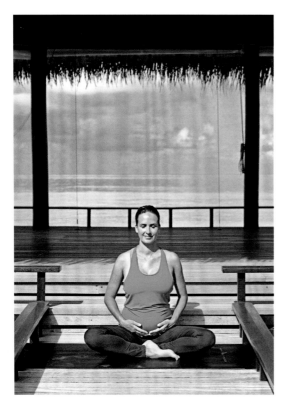

*top tip

Have sex, if you feel like it. As long as your doctor or midwife say it's OK and your pregnancy has been complication-free, sex in the last trimester can help you and your partner bond and, in the last days of pregnancy, it can even help bring on labour. However, if you don't feel like it or feel self-conscious about your bump, find other ways of being intimate, like massage or cuddling.

Meditation

Sitting in a comfortable position, using support if needed, scan your body for any tension and make sure you are as relaxed as possible.

Bring your hands on to your belly, cradling your baby. Close your eyes and open your inner eyes and look down your spinal column to your womb world where you will find your baby attached to you by the umbilical cord, growing beautifully and healthily. Become aware of your breath, your heartbeat and how strong your body is, providing everything your baby needs. Sit quietly for a while, sending love to your baby and feeling the love back, knowing you are going to be the best mummy for this baby that is taking birth through you, blessing yourself, your body, your baby, your partner and your new family unit.

FEEDING PREP

Get your feeding kit ready. If you're planning to breastfeed, make sure you have a few feeding bras and some clothes that allow easy breast access. Special breastfeeding tops are great, but stretchy cotton maxi-dresses you can pull down to expose a breast work just fine too. And get a few vest tops as well; you can wear them alone in warm weather or under regular tops in colder weather. When you pull up your regular top the vest top will stop you fully exposing yourself, and then you can pull down the vest top to feed baby. Also buy breast pads to avoid milk leaking on to your bra, and nipple cream, in case your nipples become sore. If you're planning to bottle feed, make sure you have a steriliser, formula and plenty of bottles (you'll go through six or more a day in the early days).

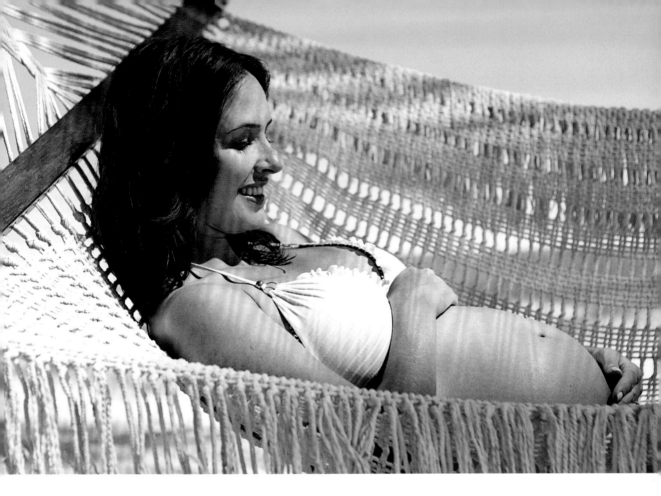

HOW TO PREPARE

The last few weeks, as your due date approaches, can be a nervewracking time, so it really helps if you feel prepared.

The support that we had was amazing and I'm so pleased that the professionals who helped us have contributed their expert advice to this book. Julie, our midwife, had a nurturing and comforting presence and we knew immediately she was the right woman to help us through the birth. She was capable, quick, calm and thoughtful and with her steady hand to guide me I helped deliver Charlotte. Similarly, Jay McGavigan, our obstetrician, was invaluable. She's one of the most respected, most highly qualified specialists in Australia

and has a fantastic bedside manner. She made Christiane and I feel so comfortable and confident throughout the pregnancy and we always knew we were in safe hands.

*top tip

Don't worry! As long as you have loved ones around you, nappies, sleepsuits and somewhere for baby to sleep, you're fine. So stop fretting about the nursery and having the right pram – you can buy things as you go along and everything will just fall into place. I promise.

THE LAST FEW WEEKS OF PREGNANCY

by Dr. C Jay McGavigan, MBBS, MD, MRCOG, FRANZCOG, obstetrician

'The last few weeks of a pregnancy are a time of great change as the body prepares for labour. You may notice your joints ache a little (more so if this is your second or third pregnancy). This is because your ligaments have started to soften and relax to enable your pelvis to expand during labour and help baby negotiate its way out.

'Throughout most of your pregnancy, your cervix is closed, holding the baby inside your uterus. As you reach the end, hormones start to soften and thin – or "ripen" – the cervix, preparing it for labour. Much of the work of labour is in opening the cervix to the passage of your baby. However, your cervix may begin to soften, thin and open even before labour begins. This varies from woman to woman, and from pregnancy to pregnancy. Some women may have a closed cervix until labour starts. Others may have pre-labour contractions that dilate their cervix to 2–3cm (or even more) before active labour actually begins.

'Your baby may begin moving lower in the pelvis, which is called engagement. You might notice this as increasing pressure in your lower abdomen and your family or friends may comment that you look different, or that your baby "has dropped". Not long before starting labour you may have a "show". This is the loss of the mucous plug that has been inside the cervix during your pregnancy, and as the cervix begins to soften and open, this plug loosens and may pass from the vagina. A show can be clear, old brown or brighter blood mixed with mucous. Some women may actually notice an increased discharge for a few days (or even weeks) before labour begins; others may not notice anything at all.

'Pre-labour contractions are known as Braxton-Hicks contractions; they're not as painful as regular ones and can be irregular. Changing activity might cause the contractions to go away or occur more often. You might experience them for several hours before they subside, or you might have them on and off for several days. The best way to deal with Braxton-Hicks is to rest as much as possible. Position changes, warm baths or showers and massage can help.'

BIRTH

'Preparation for holistic childbirth begins before you actually conceive. By optimising your health you directly optimise your baby's. Birthing is an extremely empowering experience, but, like all good things, it requires groundwork.

'I strongly encourage all my patients to enrol in childbirth education classes. They cover everything from what to expect in labour; pain relief options; assisted delivery (including forceps, vacuum or Caesarean Section); feeding (breast as well as bottle); even how to bath a baby. Make sure you ask questions – and remember there is no such thing as a stupid question. The better prepared you are, the more empowered you will be during your labour.

'Arm yourself with several techniques to manage pain during labour, such as self-hypnosis, position changes, heat packs and different breathing methods. Bring music to play for relaxation. Choose the kind of surroundings you wish to labour in: some women prefer a dark, quiet environment; others may prefer loud music. Either way, personalise your environment with little touches: a favourite pillow, a pair of socks or soothing scent – some women find lavender aromatherapy oil very soothing in labour. Remember, this is your labour and you are in control.

*top tip

Have help on standby. If you already have a child, or your partner works away a lot, make sure you have people around you whom you can call on when you go into labour.

'Try to be as mobile as you can during labour – let gravity help bring that baby out. Upright positions, such as standing, pacing around, kneeling, slow dancing, sitting and squatting, allow gravity to help move the baby down and out. Water is very soothing and many women enjoy a warm bath in early labour – standing under a warm shower is just as good.

'At the end of the day – as obstetricians, midwives and parents – we're all after the same result: a healthy mum and a healthy baby. Whether you have a natural birth or a Caesarean section, whether you hypno-birth or have an epidural, it doesn't really matter. The process is an empowering adventure and not to be feared. Fear can be alleviated by education and preparation – it's that simple.'

*top tip

Try not to make plans that involve being too far from home in the last few weeks of pregnancy. If you go somewhere – and especially if you stay overnight – take your hospital bag and notes with you just in case you go into labour.

ENSURE YOU GET EMOTIONAL SUPPORT

While the birth of a child is generally a happy, anticipated event, it's also stressful. There are so many things you may start to worry about, like how you or your partner will care for a child, what kind of parents you'll be, how your other children will react to the new baby or if you can afford a child. You might think about how the birth of a child means a loss of control over your body and your time. You might worry about your career or feel guilt about having to leave your child to return to work. All of these are stressful, so it's helpful to have frank discussions with your partner about what both of you think you'll need from each other, from other family members and from friends. If handling stress is difficult for you, or if you've had a history of depression, this might be a good time to seek therapy to help manage stress.

PREPARING FOR BIRTH

by Julie Schiller, midwife with 35 years' experience

'Many women find regular hydrotherapy, aqua classes, Pilates, yoga, stretching, meditation, massage or acupuncture helps to aid relaxation, settles their thoughts and also enhances sleep. Meeting up with like-minded friends, family or other antenatal groups can offer support to enhance feelings of relaxation and an acceptance of the life journey ahead. Writing a birth plan (this isn't a rigid perfect birth scenario, more a chance for you to think about pain relief and where you give birth) can be helpful. For example, you may want to avoid having an episiotomy (a cut between the vagina and anus), or want encouragement to move freely in labour and to try different positions, or use water, or have skin-to-skin contact with your baby immediately after the birth. Discussing these things with your midwife, doctor and partner in the weeks leading up to labour can make you less apprehensive.'

How will I know when I'm in labour?

'You need a lot of patience in the last few weeks. Things will happen in good time and it can be difficult to pinpoint exactly when labour may start, but subtle signs your baby is on the way include energetic cleaning or organisational bursts, known as "nesting", an increase in vaginal discharge, nausea, looser bowel movements and Braxton-Hicks contractions (see p. 118). Certain signs are regular, painful contractions that increase in duration, frequency and strength. You may also have a "show", which is the mucus plug coming away from your cervix which can happen in the days leading up to labour. In the absence of contractions it's not a reliable indicator that labour has started; however, with contractions it probably signifies labour has begun.

'For some women, their membranes rupture (in other words, their waters break) before they have any contractions. For others, this happens during labour or even just before they give birth. It's important to contact the midwife or place of birth when your waters break. The liquid should be a clear or whitish to pink colour and the amount can vary from a trickle to a gush. If the water is green or brown, this may indicate the baby has had a bowel movement in utero (a "meconium"), which can be dangerous if left untreated.'

What if you're overdue?

'Most women have ultrasounds now to confirm when their baby is due and are given an estimated due date, but it's just that, estimated. Babies don't often come on this date, with most being born in the days either side and up to two weeks after. So this is a time of patience! Unless your midwife or doctor says otherwise, it's safe to wait as early induction can lead to a cascade of intervention such as more pain relief, monitoring, instrumental births (for example, with the use of forceps) and even a C-section.

'Some women prepare for labour with acupuncture, where the practitioner performs a ripening of the cervix over several sessions. Some midwives offer a stretch and sweep, which is a vaginal examination that can stimulate the release of prostaglandins if the cervix is already starting to open up. Walking and staying upright so the baby is encouraged to move down into the pelvis and put pressure on the cervix to help it soften and efface (shorten) can help if you have the energy. Sexual intercourse, including ejaculation of sperm, can help the release of prostaglandins that help ripen the cervix and stimulate contractions, as can nipple stimulation. Curry and other spicy foods can stimulate the bowel which is next to the uterus, also stimulating contractions. Never take castor oil (this used to be recommended) as it can have a violent, very unpleasant effect. Not only does it empty the bowel but it can also have a disastrous and distressing effect on the foetus if labour is stimulated so violently.'

The stages of labour

'There are different stages of labour and each stage can last days, hours or minutes. It's different for each woman and each birth. Here are the different stages you'll go through...

Pre-labour/latent stage: As the body prepares for labour, the cervix, which is generally long and firm, begins to soften, thin (efface) and open (dilate), as well as move from a posterior position (pointing slightly towards the back) to a mid-anterior position (more towards the front). Not every woman is aware of this stage happening but there may be a few subtle signs (see left). This phase is sometimes referred to as 'pre-labour' and it is important to stay rested and well hydrated as you wait for labour to establish.

Early labour: When your contractions become regular you're officially in early labour. Unlike with Braxton Hicks, during early labour your contractions will become longer, stronger and closer together. This stage ends when your cervix is dilated to 4cm and at this point they'll be every 5 minutes and will last up to 60 seconds. You should be able to cope with early labour at home – remember, walking around helps the baby shift into the right position for birth. However, early contractions can still be painful and breathing through them or warm baths can help.

The first stage: Known as active labour, this is when your contractions become longer, closer together and more intense. During this stage your cervix will dilate from 4 to 8cm. If you're giving birth in hospital, now's the time to go in. You probably won't be able to talk through your contractions anymore and, if you decide it's right for you, now is the time to ask for pain relief. If this is your first baby, active labour can last up to 24 hours. However, it can also last as little as one hour. If you can cope, moving around during this stage helps – but you may have to stop during a contraction. Rocking on a birthing ball or trying out different positions will also help.

The transition stage: When your cervix goes from 8 to 10cm (fully dilated), it's known as the transitional phase. This is the most intense part of labour and is often the time many women feel like they can't go on – but trust us, you can! Your baby is bearing down and you may feel like pushing but the important thing is not to do so until you are fully dilated as otherwise the cervix can become swollen and bruised. You may start to grunt, groan and feel detached from what's going on around you. This stage can last minutes or hours – it's usually quicker with second and third babies, but every woman is different.

The second stage: Otherwise known as the pushing stage, this is when you begin to push your baby out. You'll be encouraged to push during each contraction, and rest in between so you build up strength for your next contraction/push. Upright positions, kneeling and being on all fours can all aid the descent of the baby. Eventually your baby will "crown" – which means the midwife will be able to see the top of its head and some women like to use a mirror so they can see it too. You may feel a burning or stinging sensation as the skin around your vagina stretches to its full capacity. Your midwife will encourage you to slow down pushing at this point and to breathe and pant your way through this next part to reduce tearing. Once the head is out, your midwife will ensure the cord isn't round its neck and may suction his/her nose and mouth. Then with one – or a few more – pushes the rest of your baby's body will be born and, as soon as possible, placed on your chest for skin-to-skin warmth and bonding. If it is a water birth, the baby won't breathe until it is brought into the air. Like the rest of labour, the pushing stage varies from woman to woman but as a general rule it's quicker with subsequent babies.

The third stage: This involves pushing out the placenta. Your uterus will start to contract again and your placenta will detach from the wall of your uterus. It is usually painless and happens from 5 minutes and up to an hour after birth. You may be asked to push and you may be given an injection to help it come out. The midwife and birth attendants will be vigilant in observing this is expelled effectively and will then inspect the vagina and perineum and perform any stitching that is necessary.'

After the birth

'Skin-to-skin contact and breastfeeding are recommended as soon as possible to help relax both mum and baby and encourage bonding and the release of the feel-good hormone oxytocin. A shower after childbirth is probably the nicest shower you will ever have, washing away the body's aches and tiredness. Nestling into a clean bed, then, to eat, drink and snuggle with your baby is blissful. Keep things simple with your partner and let visitors wait for a few hours – unless you want them there. An ice pack wrapped inside a perineal pad can ease the discomfort, swelling and any bruising. Some women take Arnica, which can help with bruising. Emptying the bladder after birth is also important. Some stinging may occur which can be eased by going in the shower or splashing water over the perineum.'

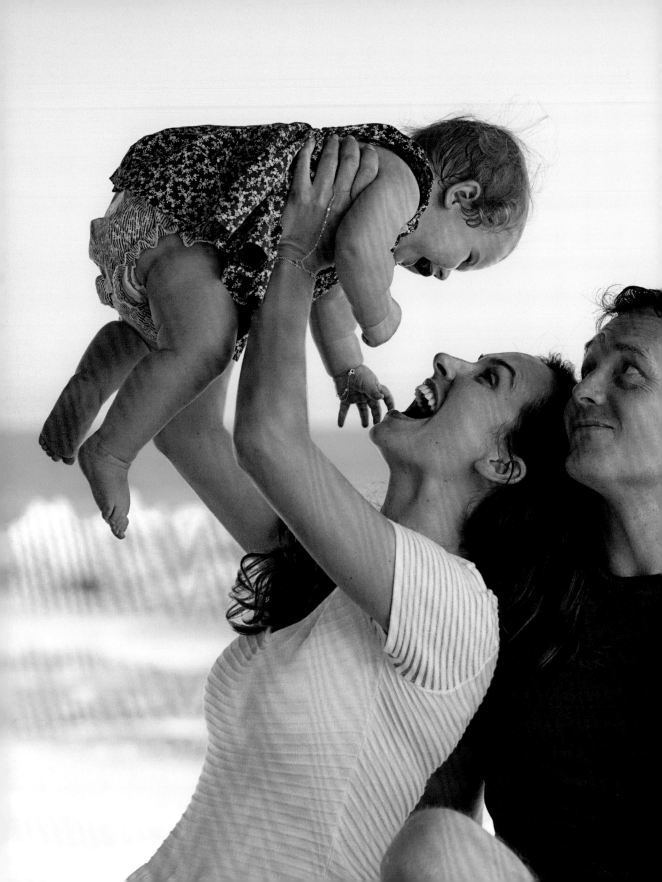

CHAPTER 6

THE SURVIVAL GUIDE FOR NEW MUMS

A NEW BABY

Congratulations, you amazing miracle mama! Life is different now in ways you could never have imagined. Your little baby is here and needs you for everything. It is an overwhelming responsibility – but you can do this; just believe in yourself and fill every moment with as much love and confidence as you can. The thing to remember is that there is no right or wrong way to feel, and whatever you are feeling – scared, excited, full of love, exhausted, bored, lonely or all of the above and more – is normal.

Ask most mums and they'll tell you that life post-birth is a hazy blur of loveliness... most of the time. But it's also a physically and emotionally challenging time and you need to take care of yourself more than ever in the weeks after childbirth. In fact, think of it as the 'fourth trimester' – another 12 weeks of development for you and your baby.

Too many mums forget about themselves the moment they give birth and just focus on their baby. The baby gets fed the best (whether it's breast or formula milk) and their every need is catered for. Whereas poor mum often lives on coffee and sugar and very little sleep. But it's vital you take as good care of yourself as you do your baby (or at least try to).

Your body has just carried you and your baby through nine months of pregnancy and the enormous challenge of labour. Christiane is and always will be my hero for this – witnessing her strength and courage during childbirth is something that will stay with me for ever. Whether you had a quick, uncomplicated birth, a Caesarean or a long and difficult labour, childbirth takes an enormous amount out of you. And now you have your baby in your arms the journey has only just begun, as you embark upon weeks and months of sleepless nights, constant feeds and endless nappy changes. Add to this the stream of visitors who will want to come and see your new baby and, if you're already a mum, the demands of your other children and of running a home. Being a mum is amazing and beautiful, but it's also tough and relentless and I am in awe of every single one of you.

So in this chapter I'm going to give you the Clean & Lean new mum survival guide; and Maria Lally – the genius who helps me write the Clean & Lean books, and who has had two babies while doing so – will also share her own experiences. I'm going to cover everything from how you should eat in the early weeks, to foods that boost your milk supply, the two-minute magical meditation, how to benefit most from the little sleep you get and how to begin the (very gentle) road to getting your body back.

*top tip

Rest when your baby rests. Don't be tempted to rush around, catching up on the housework.

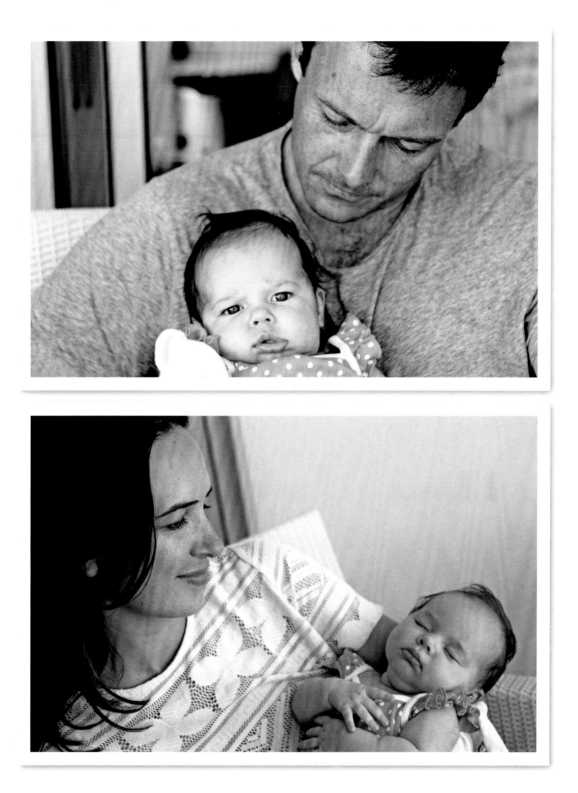

YOUR POST-CHILDBIRTH DIET

Whether you breastfeed or not, you don't have to make any huge changes to the way you eat during this time. It's just important to follow a balanced Clean & Lean diet that includes wholegrains, fruits, vegetables, lean proteins, eggs and dairy. If you are breastfeeding, it's often recommended that you increase your calorie intake by around 400–500 a day. However, advice varies and depends on your pre-pregnancy weight and how much you gained during pregnancy, as well as how active you are. Mother Nature is very clever at drawing on maternal fat stores so, in practice, only half of these extra calories may be required. Therefore the best advice is, as always, listen to your body: if you feel hungry, eat. Extreme dieting will ruin your body, affect your milk supply, slow down your recovery and make you feel even more tired. But foods full of nutrients will have the opposite effect, so think Clean & Lean, not calories.

Make sure you drink plenty of water too. You need plenty of extra fluid to allow for all the fluid you lose in breast milk. Furthermore, during breastfeeding, your body produces the hormone oxytocin which can make you feel thirsty, so always keep a big glass of water close by and one next to your bed – if you wake in the night to feed your baby, it will be right there for you. There are currently no safe guidelines on caffeine consumption while breastfeeding, but it's best to limit yourself to what you were having during pregnancy (see p. 14). There are plenty of good reasons for limiting caffeine – for a start, it can cause your baby to struggle to fall asleep and it's also a diuretic, so it can cause dehydration and even more trips to the toilet.

As for alcohol, studies show that the occasional drink is unlikely to harm your breastfed baby, so a small glass of Champagne when you come out of hospital to toast the newborn won't do much harm. Any more might be risky, though, as it could pass into your milk supply, and because new babies feed little and often, your body won't have the chance to process the alcohol before baby's next feed. Alcohol can also reduce your milk supply and, as I explained on p. 15, it also makes you feel tired and causes weight gain, so I'd advise avoiding it altogether.

Absolutely don't smoke during this time. Even if you do it away from your baby, they'll be exposed to nicotine through your breast milk or via your clothes and hair. If you're struggling to give up cigarettes, speak to your doctor immediately. And tell your partner, friends and family that they can't smoke around you or your baby either.

Lastly, take a good postnatal supplement that contains vitamin D (most do) – babies need this for strong bones and teeth and, as sunlight is the best source of vitamin D and not everybody gets enough every day, new mums should take it in supplement form.

SNACKS TO KEEP AROUND THE HOUSE

* Bags of raw, unsalted nuts
* Whole fruit
* Vegetables (go for easy things that don't need peeling, like cherry tomatoes, cucumber, peppers and sugar-snap peas)
* Pots of hummus and homemade guacamole
* Oatcakes and rye crackers (with nut butter or hummus)
* Full-fat natural Greek yogurt
* Full-fat organic milk (good-quality breast milk requires double the usual daily recommended calcium intake)

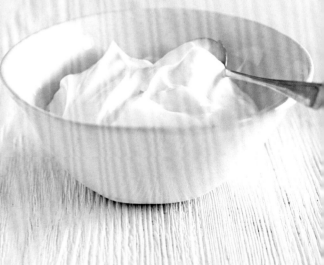

POST-BIRTH

by Julie Schiller, midwife

'Rejoice in the fact that your amazing body has just birthed your baby! Immediately after the birth you may look about five or six months pregnant. Your uterus (womb) will go down over the next six weeks. Post-birth bleeding (lochia) will be like a heavy period for the first few days and will then slow down and start to settle to a lighter colour within the week. Some women bleed for up to six weeks, others finish at two weeks.

'If this is your second baby, you may experience after-pains which are contraction-like, especially during feeding. Hot packs, such as a hot-water bottle, or simple pain relief can help to ease the discomfort as the uterus contracts back down. In the days following birth you'll pass urine in greater volume (as opposed to the small, frequent dribbles you had before!). Therefore any fluid retained usually improves.

'It may be a couple of days before you have a bowel movement after the birth. Eat nourishing food, high in fibre, and drink plenty of water so your first bowel movement isn't too firm or difficult to pass... especially if your stitches are painful.

Breastfeeding

'Breastfeeding is one of the most natural things in the world, but that doesn't mean it comes easily to everyone and many women have problems, which can cause them to give up in the first few weeks. And while it's every woman's right to feed her baby however she feels is best for her and baby, if you do want to breastfeed but experience any of the following difficulties, here's how you can overcome them.

A reluctant feeder: A newborn's instinct to breastfeed is usually very strong –however, some babies are very sleepy after birth and reluctant to feed. Skin-to-skin contact, gently brushing your baby's mouth or nose with your nipple and feeding on demand will help. If you're worried, speak to your midwife.

Sore nipples: In the early days and weeks, your nipples may become dry, cracked or start to bleed. If you experience discomfort during a feed, slide your little finger gently into the corner of baby's mouth until they come away. Pain can often be due to a poor latch, so ask your health visitor or midwife for advice immediately. In the mean time, you can help yourself by using a good nipple cream containing lanolin, squeezing out a few drops of breast milk and rubbing it gently into the sore area, wearing a cotton bra or even better, letting the air get to your breasts if you're at home.

Engorged or painful breasts: Sometimes your breasts may become swollen, hard or sore – especially in the first week as your milk comes in. Drink plenty of water and feed on demand. However, after the first week if your baby isn't latching on properly they may not be draining your breast at each feed which can cause engorgement. Missing a feed – for example, if you're supplementing with formula – or wearing a too tight bra can also cause problems. So wear a well fitted cotton bra and try placing a chilled cabbage leaf in the cups. Once feeding is established, engorgement should improve.

Mastitis: If engorgement doesn't go away or a milk duct becomes blocked it's important to treat it as soon as possible to prevent mastitis (an inflammation of the breast). Symptoms include a warm or tender breast, a red patch on the breast, flu-like symptoms and a temperature. Carry on breastfeeding and seek help immediately from your midwife, health visitor or doctor, who may give you antibiotics. In the meantime, keep feeding (especially from the tender breast) while gently massaging the sore area towards the nipple, drink plenty of water and hand express. Try doing this in a warm bath or shower and massage the area around your sore breast. Lastly, rest as much as possible.

Low milk supply: Many new mums worry they're not producing enough milk for their baby, but chances are they are. Signs you're producing enough include your baby gaining weight, seeming well and producing wet nappies throughout the day. A stressful birth, dummies and formula feeds can sometimes reduce milk in the early days, as can trying to put your baby on a feeding schedule. In the early weeks your baby needs to be on the breast as often as they want to build up your milk supply. Resting when you can, drinking plenty of water and eating a healthy balanced diet can help your milk supply. Speak to your midwife or health visitor if you continue to be concerned.'

HOW TO SLEEP LIKE A BABY

Sleep is a big part of my Clean & Lean regime – it helps keep your body strong and healthy, your metabolism fired up and it makes you mentally alert and less stressed.

If this is your first baby, your new sleep routine will be a huge shock. A recent study found that parents miss out on six whole months' worth of sleep in the first two years of their baby's life. Among other things, a lack of sleep can cause hunger and sugar cravings. However, it's tough to sleep properly when you have a new baby. And while I can't wave a magic sleep wand over you and your baby, I can help you make sure that the sleep you do get it as restorative as possible.

Newborns often sleep for up to 17 hours in a 24-hour period, having used up a lot of energy and effort being born and with high levels of the sleep hormone melatonin in their system as it crosses the placenta. So try to take advantage of this, and while it's tempting to invite friends and family round every moment of the first week, try to limit their visits. Once important family members have met the new arrival, ask others to wait a while. People will understand, and if they don't, that's tough. This is your time to recover from the birth, bond with your precious baby and spend time as a new family with your partner. So, rather than rushing around making drinks and meals for visitors or doing housework, just rest when your baby rests. Don't worry about replying to congratulation texts or thanking people for presents or flowers because you're going to need your energy in the weeks ahead.

Your little one may lull you into a false sense of security at first and you may think you have a great sleeper on your hands, but by day seven, levels of melatonin will disappear, so expect a more wakeful baby after that. They'll still be sleeping a lot, but they'll be waking around the clock for feeds and comfort. As the months go by, the baby won't fall asleep straight after each feed – they'll have more awake time and may need settling to sleep. So get used to sleeping like your baby and rest when they do. If you can't switch off (lots of new mums are hardwired to listening out for their baby's cries and struggle to sleep when they get the chance), lie down on the sofa and rest with a book. While this isn't as restorative as actual sleep it will help

your body to feel rejuvenated. This is also a good reason to limit coffee in the exhausting first few weeks; if you drink a couple of coffees in the morning, you'll be too wired to sleep during your baby's morning nap.

SWADDLING

This is a wrapping technique that creates a slight pressure around your baby's body, so they feel like they're still in the womb. Here's how to do it safely:

✳ Spread out a cot sheet or cellular blanket and fold in half to make a triangle.

✳ Lay your baby on their back with their neck on the centre of the fold and their feet facing the point.

✳ Pull one top corner across the baby's body and tuck it under the opposite arm. Pull the bottom point up and under the baby, folding it back, if necessary, so you don't cover the face.

✳ Hold your baby's free arm against them, then pull the other corner of the blanket firmly over their body before tucking it under their back.

✳ Make sure your baby is comfortable and can breathe easily.

*top tip
Learning to be a parent takes time. The transition can be easier than you expect, or more overwhelming than you ever imagined, but it's an amazing, rewarding, mindblowing, once-in-a-lifetime experience to embrace as a privilege. Good luck!

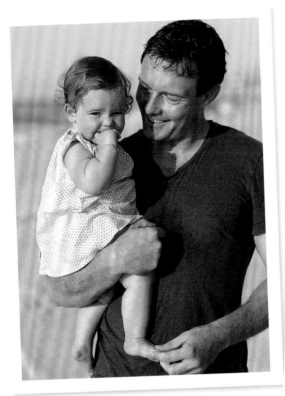

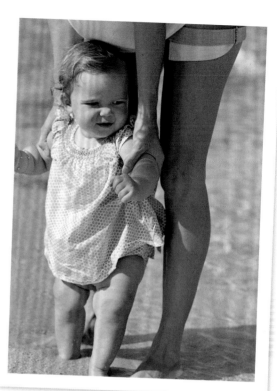

HELPING YOUR BABY TO SLEEP

Most new mums ask: how can I help my baby sleep better? In the early weeks it's hard to establish any kind of routine as baby's sleeping patterns are erratic and they feed and sleep little and often. However, it's never too early to nudge them gently towards a routine, and here's how:

Get into the bathtime habit

Babies don't really need a bath in the first couple of weeks. However, studies show that warm water stimulates the production of melatonin in a baby's brain and induces sleep. So, after about a month, it's a good idea to make bathtime a bedtime ritual which your baby will learn to associate with sleep.

Keep your baby warm (but not too hot)

Your baby can't regulate their own body temperature very well, so make sure their bedroom is warm enough (especially for winter babies). A thermometer helps – aim for around 16–20°C, but use your common sense: does the temperature in the room feel OK to you? Could you sleep in there?

Sing to your baby

Studies show that when babies hear singing it lowers their heart rate and calms them down. Familiar noises also help release the relaxing hormone oxytocin which can help babies settle. It can also help to say 'Sshhh' repeatedly – they will have heard your blood swishing around to the pattern of your heartbeat when they were in the womb, so saying the 'Ssshh, ssshh, ssshh' sound will comfort them at nap- or bedtime.

Set the scene

Don't fill your baby's room with lots of brightly coloured, noisy toys. You want their room to provide a calm, soothing environment that helps – not hinders – sleep. Invest in blackout blinds or a blackout lining for nap- and bedtimes, as darkness helps your baby distinguish between night and day and will help them to sleep better.

OTHER TIPS ON SURVIVING THE DAY AS A NEW MUM

✳ **Forget the housework.** Seriously, just forget it. This can be especially hard if you're house-proud, but in the first few weeks of having a new baby, don't worry about the chores. Do the bare minimum (or, better still, get somebody else to do it) and worry about it later when life is a bit calmer.

✳ **Ask for help.** When visitors come to see you, ask them to bring food and drink. Don't feel bad about this – people want to be useful. Practical help from family and friends is also vital, like providing childcare and support. Remember the old saying, 'It takes a village to bring up a child.'

✳ **Don't let visitors hog your baby.** Don't let visitors sit and cuddle your sleeping baby while you rush around making them tea – unless you want a break from holding your baby for a while, which is also normal.

✳ **Know it's OK to cry.** The first few weeks of new motherhood can be very overwhelming. Even if you're over the moon at becoming a parent and completely in love with your new baby, it's normal to feel overcome at times. It's often due to tiredness, hormones or just the huge life changes you're undergoing. So if you feel sad, cry. It's important for many women to talk through their birthing experience, especially if it's been traumatic, or different from how they imagined it, so talk about it to your partner and midwife and remember it's OK. However, if you feel tearful most days, speak to your midwife, as it could be an early sign of postnatal depression. If it is, this is extremely common, and there's plenty of help out there.

✳ **Don't feel bad about being 'rude'.** If a friend is due round and you're exhausted having been up all night with the baby, cancel their visit. If visitors have outstayed their welcome and you're desperate for them to go so you can rest, tell them.

✳ **Don't try to be Superwoman.** If your mother-in-law offers to do your ironing, don't be polite – let her do it. If your friend offers to take baby for a walk, while you take a bath or have a nap, say yes.

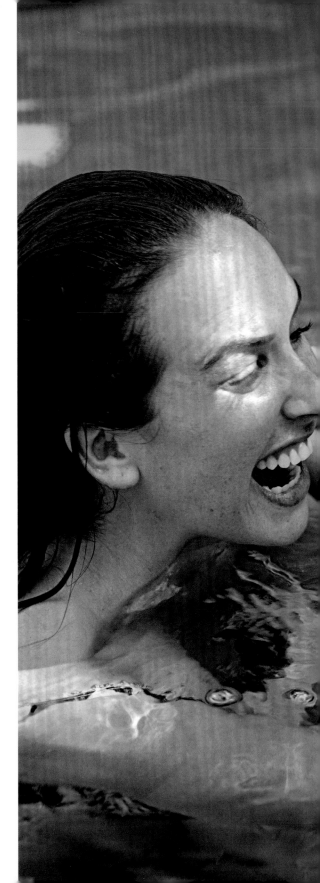

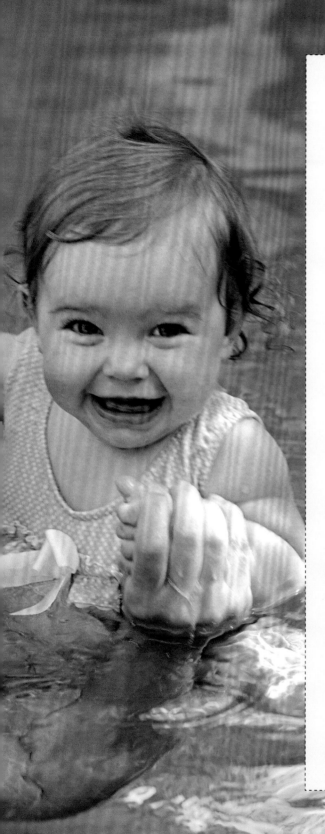

MARIA'S STORY

'Nothing – and I mean nothing – prepares you for the first few months of first-time motherhood. When I became pregnant with my daughter Sophia in 2010 I'd enjoyed a busy and deadline-driven career as a health journalist in London for almost ten years. I was working on a glossy magazine by day and working on the first *Clean & Lean* book by night. Nothing phased me and I felt confident about the challenges of having a baby. How hard could it be, I remember thinking.

'However, when Sophia was born, a baby sized bomb went off in my lovely, calm, organised life. Sophia – quite rightly – demanded every last ounce of my time, love, strength and energy. I felt tiredness like I'd never thought possible. It was bone-numbing. I had a long labour and was already two days behind on sleep when I suddenly had a new baby to care for.

'Like all good health journalists, I used to snack on avocado and oatcakes, or seeds and fruit. But suddenly, I craved endless cups of coffee, buttered toast and chocolate bars because that's all I had time to eat and I needed that sugar hit. However, I quickly realised this way of eating just makes you feel even more tired, so I went for quick and easy Clean & Lean options like omelettes, fruit, chopped vegetables and lots of oatcakes and rye crackers. After about six weeks I took Sophia for long walks every day, but I didn't feel bad if I fancied an afternoon on the sofa either. I didn't think about calories or exercise, and I tried not to worry about my jiggling stomach or wider hips (don't worry – they go back to normal in time). After about six months I was back in all my old clothes and by about ten months I was even a bit slimmer, thanks to endlessly chasing around after a then-crawling Sophia.

'Four months ago I had another beautiful daughter, Rosie, and it's now double the workload, but twice the fun. It's easier second time around because that first year of first-time motherhood toughens you up and makes you more resilient than you ever realised you could be. I think all mums should congratulate themselves on making it through each day, as motherhood is relentless. But it's worth it and we wouldn't have it any other way, would we?'

by Maria Lally, co-author of *Clean & Lean* books

6-WEEK POST-BABY EXERCISES

After about six weeks, if you feel up to it, you've had your six-week check-up with your doctor and all is well, you can increase the duration of your walks, as well as your effort level. But ensure that you listen to your body and don't push yourself.

Six weeks is the perfect point to begin to spend more time with your baby outdoors – your partner will probably have gone back to work, the constant stream of visitors you had in the early weeks will have slowed down and you'll probably feel like getting out of the house. It's good for your baby too – fresh air helps to stimulate them, the change of scenery often stops them from becoming restless and crying and the gently rocking motion of the pram also induces sleep.

Pushing a pram is a great workout in itself, so try to head out for a walk at least once a day. If you feel up to it, start to increase the duration of your walks and slowly build up to 45 minutes or an hour 3–4 times a week (or, ideally, every day). Try incorporating a gentle incline into your walks, being sure not to push yourself too hard. Walking with a pram works your glutes (bottom), hamstrings, abdominals and pelvic-floor muscles. The combination will create a long, lean profile and a perkier, firmer bottom.

As well as pram-walking, here are some other exercises you can start to do after six weeks. Try to perform this workout 2–4 times a week on non-consecutive days. However, listen to your body and, if you feel tired, don't fight it. Do what you can – 2 workouts a week is great, 4 is amazing and, if you do none, that is also fine, just whatever feels right to you.

*top tip

Stretching will help balance out the body from holding the baby and help blood flow to tired, tense muscles. Neck and chest stretches are very important post-pregnancy.

EXERCISE	REPS	SETS	REST
Tummy vacuum	8–10	2–3	30 secs
Superman	10–12/side	2–3	30 secs
Hip extension with mini-band	12–15/side	2–3	30 secs
Single-knee external rotation with mini-band	8–10/side	2–3	30 secs
Mini-band walking	10/side	2–3	30 secs
Y	15	2–3	30 secs
T	15	2–3	60 secs

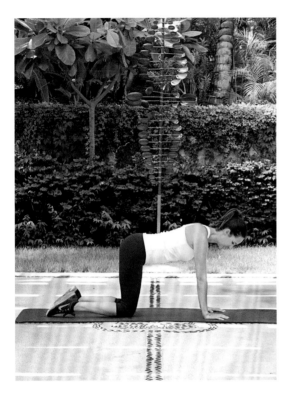

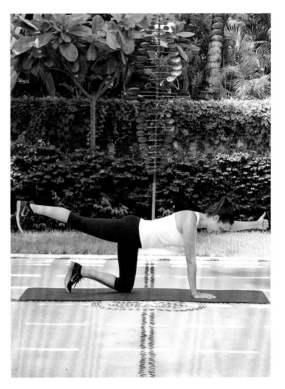

Tummy vacuum

Start position: Support yourself on your hands and knees with hands under shoulders, arms straight and knees under hips. Ensure your arms and thighs remain at right angles to the floor, keep your back straight and your head aligned with your upper back.

The movement: Relax your stomach, letting it sag towards the floor while maintaining a flat back. Then squeeze your tummy muscles and pull your belly button towards the ceiling, still maintaining a flat back, and hold for 5 seconds. Repeat 8–10 times.

Superman

Start position: Support yourself on your hands and knees with hands under shoulders and knees under hips and with your toes firmly pointed into the floor. Ensure your spine and neck are in a straight line by keeping your gaze to the floor, just in front of your fingertips.

The movement: Extend your left arm out in front of you beyond your head, thumb up, while extending your right leg backwards – imagine you are being pulled from either end. Return to the start position and repeat 10–12 times on each side.

*top tip

As you draw your belly button in, squeeze your pelvic floor muscles (that stop the flow of urine) as this aids an easier recovery.

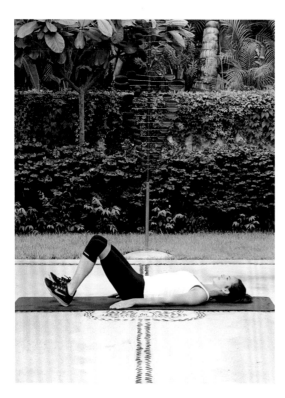
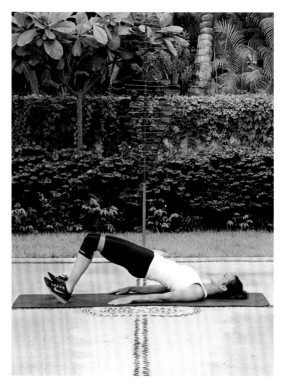

Hip extension with mini-band

Start position: Place a Bodyism mini-band of your chosen strength just above your knees. Lie on your back with both knees bent and heels on the ground. Point your toes up to the ceiling, and place your arms by your sides.

The movement: Lift your hips off the ground, raising them as high as you can go, squeezing the glutes (your butt muscles, which help protect your lower back). Pause at the top for 1 second, then return to the start position, ensuring your full back meets the floor. Repeat 10–15 times.

*top tip

This exercise will help switch on and strengthen your glute muscles, which will help to protect your lower back.

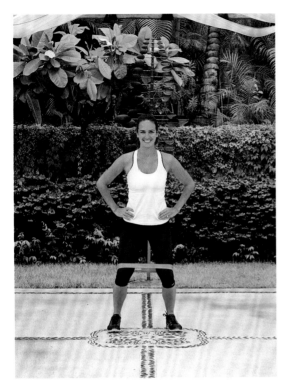
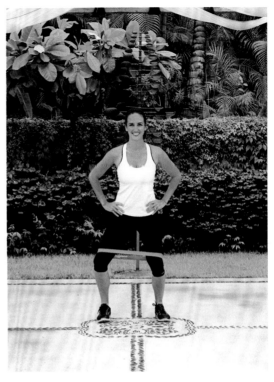

Single-knee external rotation with mini-band

Start position: Place a Bodyism mini-band of your chosen strength just above your knees. Stand with your knees bent and feet hip-width apart and pull your belly button in towards the spine to engage your core.

The movement: Keeping the soles of your feet firmly rooted to the floor, rotate one knee outwards, pushing against the mini band. Then slowly return the knee to the start position and repeat this 8–10 times on each side.

*top tip
This exercise also helps
to switch on and strengthen
your glutes.

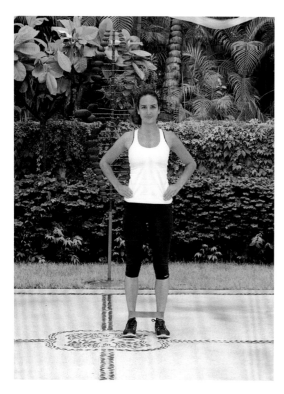
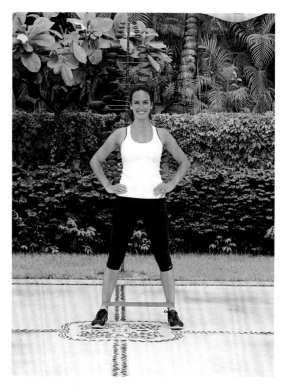

Mini-band walking

Start position: Place a Bodyism mini-band of your chosen strength just above your ankles. Stand with your feet hip-width apart, hands resting on your hips, and engage the core by pulling your belly button in towards your spine.

The movement: Take one large step out sideways to the right, keeping the legs straight and without using your body for momentum. Then bring your left foot in half a step, keeping tension in the band all the time. Repeat this movement for 10 steps on each side.

*top tip

This exercise lifts your bottom like nothing else. Creating long, lean, beautiful muscles in your upper legs, it also helps stabilise your hip, knee and ankle joints by strengthening the glutes.

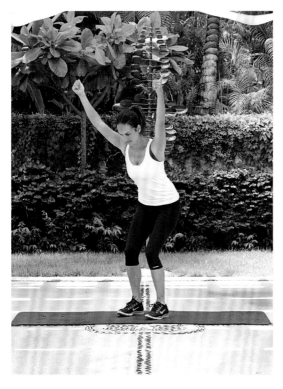

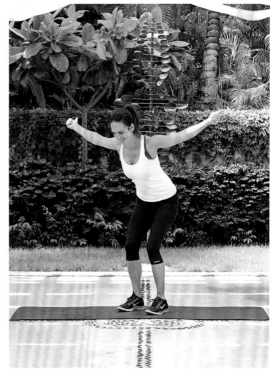

Y

T

Start position: Stand with your feet hip-width apart, bend your knees and stick your bottom out, so your upper body leans forwards 45 degrees. Hold your hands directly below your chest with fists clenched and thumbs up, keeping your head and back in a straight line, your shoulders back and down. Engage your core by pulling your belly button in towards the spine.

The movement: Raise both hands to create a 'Y' shape above your head with your arms by your ears, then return to the starting point. Repeat 15 times.

Start position: Stand with your feet hip-width apart. Bend your knees and lean forwards so your torso is at a 45-degree angle. Keep your head and back in a straight line, your shoulders back and down and your hands directly below your chest with fists clenched and thumbs pointing outwards. Engage your core by pulling your belly button in towards the spine.

The movement: Keeping your body still and your core engaged, raise your arms out to the side to form a 'T' shape, then return to the start position. Repeat 15 times.

*top tip

These exercises are designed to help strengthen your upper back, the key area that provides support when holding your baby.

12-WEEK POST-BABY EXERCISES

After about twelve weeks you can gently step up your exercise routine, but as always, only if you feel up to it. So now is the time you can make your walks a little longer, your pace a little brisker and you can incorporate some new moves into your routine like the ones below, especially if you had a straightforward birth and pregnancy. If you had a Caesarean, an episiotomy or any stitches or other problems associated with the birth, speak to your GP, health visitor or midwife to ensure you're healing properly before embarking on any exercise.

By around 12 weeks, tiredness may be creeping in, so don't push yourself too hard. See exercise as a way of giving you more energy – not something that's going to make you even more exhausted. So keep your workouts brief and try to do them in the fresh air or with a friend so they energise you and improve your mood. Try to get somebody to look after your baby while you do them, rather than rushing through them during baby's naptime.

Make sure you're eating a well-balanced diet alongside your workouts and stay hydrated – especially if you're breastfeeding. Remember, don't cut calories, just eat Clean & Lean.

The same goes for sleep – never pick exercise over sleep, because sleep will help your body recover better from pregnancy and childbirth. If you're sleep deprived, your body won't have the energy to get you through a workout, so make sure you're well rested before you exercise.

From this point on, use the six-week programme as your warm-up, then perform the following strength programme that is designed to strengthen your posture, create a stable base and burn some fat. Aim to perform this workout 3-4 times a week on non-consecutive days. However, listen to your body do whatever feels right to you. I can't say this enough. These workouts should feel good, not put you in any pain or discomfort, so take it easy.

EXERCISE	REPS	SETS	REST
Squat with push press	12–15	2–3	30 secs
Row with towel	10–15	2–3	30 secs
Squat	12–15	2–3	30 secs
Triceps dip	8–10	2–3	30 secs
T	12–15	2–3	30 secs
Opposites	10/side	2–3	30 secs

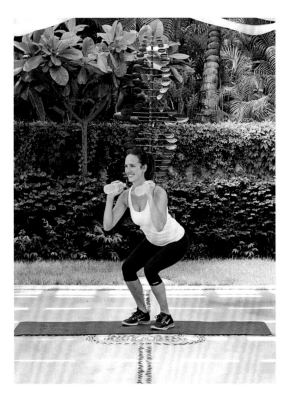
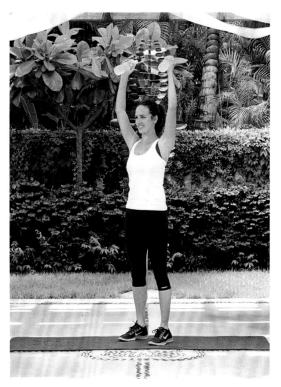

Squat with push press

Start position: Stand with hips shoulder-width apart and holding a weight, or even a large bottle of water, in each hand. Squat down, keeping your chest open, and raise your hands in front of your shoulders. Engage your core by pulling your belly button in towards the spine.

The movement: Stand up by pushing through the heels and bring the hips forwards so that the knees and hips are extended. As the hips fully extend, push the water bottles (or weights) over your head so that the arms, hips and knees are fully extended. Then slowly lower the water bottles (or weights) to the starting position and repeat 12–15 times.

*top tip
This exercise will strengthen your glutes and shoulders.

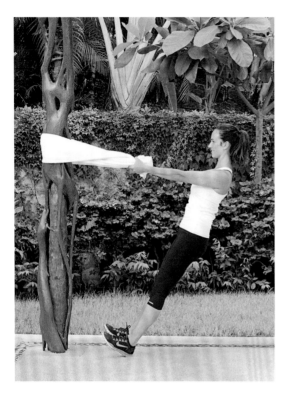 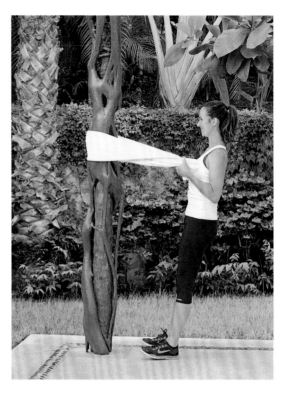

Row with towel

Start position: Wrap a towel securely around a post or narrow tree trunk. Stand near the post or tree and take the ends of the towel in your hands, then extend your arms out fully, leaning backwards. Keep the weight on your heels and a straight line from the top of your head to your heels. Engage your core by pulling your belly button in towards the spine.

The movement: Keeping your elbows tucked in, pull your body up so your hands are brought close to your chest whilst your body remains in a straight line. Return to the start position and repeat 10-15 times.

*top tip

This exercise will strengthen the back muscles that are essential to improving your posture – a key area for new mothers when carrying the baby. It is a great exercise to do outdoors.

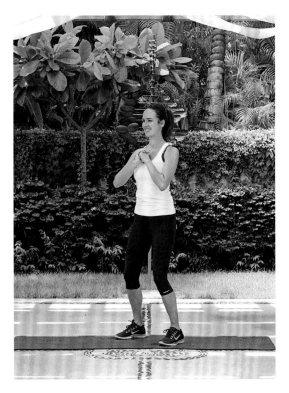
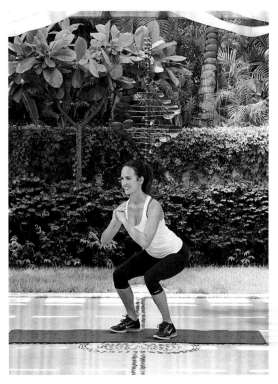

Squat

Start position: Stand with your feet hip-width apart and hands clenched in front of your chest. Engage your core by pulling your belly button in towards the spine

The movement: Keeping your hands clenched in front of your chest, squat down by pushing your hips back and bending the knees until your thighs are parallel to the floor. Throughout the movement, keep your torso upright. Return to the start position by pushing through the hips and the heels and repeat 12–15 times.

*top tip
This exercise will help strengthen your glutes, hamstrings and thighs.

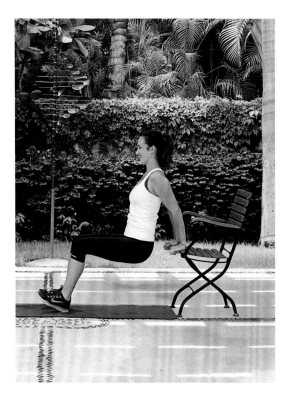
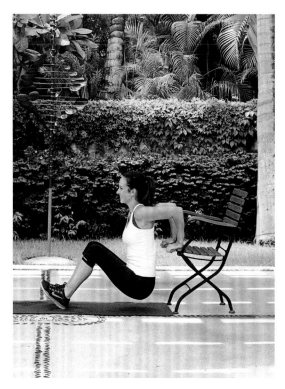

Triceps dip

Start position: Using a step/low chair/bench, sit your back and butt against the front and place your hands behind you on the edge. Keep your knees at 90 degrees, heels on the floor and toes up in the air. Lift your body up so that your hips are off the step and level with your hands. Engage your core by pulling your belly button in towards the spine.

The movement: Slowly lower yourself down towards the ground by bending the arms until your elbows are at 90 degrees. Then return to the start position by pushing your palms down on the support. Repeat 8-10 times.

*top tip

Go as low as you feel comfortable. As you become stronger, aim to lower yourself until your elbows are at 90 degrees.

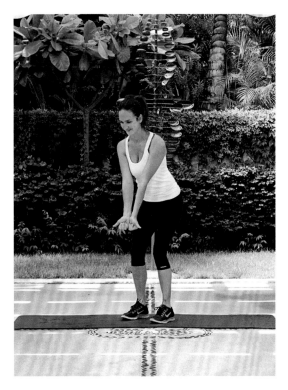
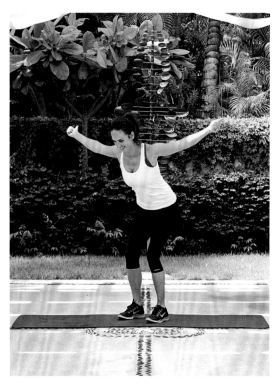

T

Start position: Stand with your feet hip-width apart. Bend your knees and lean forwards so your torso is at a 45-degree angle. Keep your head and back in a straight line, your shoulders back and down and your hands directly below your chest with fists clenched and thumbs pointing outwards. Engage your core by pulling your belly button in towards the spine.

The movement: Keeping your body still and your core engaged, raise your arms out to the side to form a 'T' shape, then return to the start position. Repeat 12–15 times.

*top tip

This is a great exercise for improving the strength of the muscles between your shoulder blades, which are essential for good posture and will help make holding your baby easier.

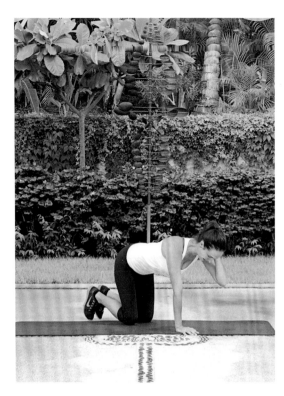 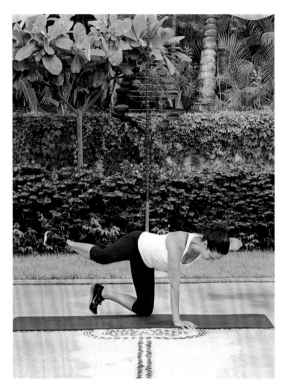

Opposites

Start position: Support yourself on your hands and knees with hands under shoulders and knees under hips. Maintain a flat back and keep your neck in a straight line with your back. Place your left hand on the base of your neck and engage your core by pulling your belly button in towards the spine.

The movement: Lift the right knee out to the side until it is level with the hip, while at the same time raising the left elbow until it is level with the left shoulder. Then slowly return the elbow and knee to the start position. Repeat 10 times on each side.

*top tip

This is an incredibly effective exercise for improving the strength of your postural muscles and lower back.

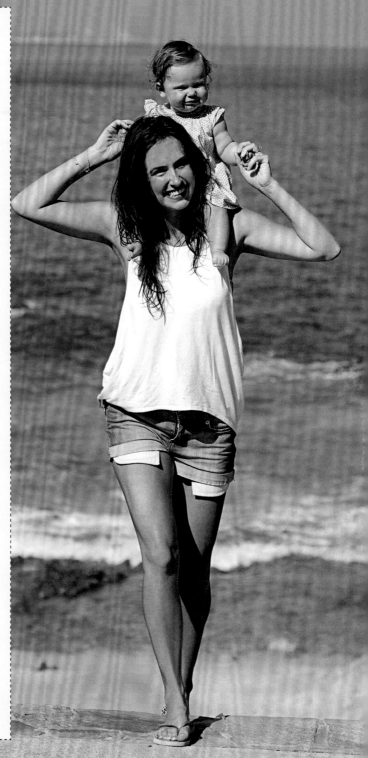

AVOID 'BABY BACK'

Many women find they have back problems some time in the first year after having a baby and 'baby back' is the term I use to describe this. Various hormones during pregnancy relax your ligaments to prepare your body for childbirth. Your abdominal muscles, which would usually help keep your spine strong and healthy, also stretch during pregnancy, making them weaker. When you then have the baby you'll carry them around a lot, and while the average baby weighs 7 or 8lb (3–4kg) at birth, they often double their birthweight in the first six months. You'll spend time with baby perched on your hip, you'll bend down to change them or put them in the car seat. Then, when the baby starts to crawl and learn to walk, you'll bend down to chase or help them. You'll also bend down numerous times throughout the day to scoop up toys. It's the perfect storm. Thankfully, however, there are plenty of ways to help yourself:

✳ Strengthen your abdominal muscles. There are lots of exercises in this chapter that will help you do this. Your abs support your spine, so once you feel up to it, do some gentle exercises to strengthen your abs which will, in turn, help to prevent lower-back pain.
✳ Bend with your knees. Don't bend down from your hips, keeping your legs straight, to pick up toys or your baby. Bend down with both your knees, keeping a straight back.
✳ Change baby on a waist-height changing table. This will help to prevent unnecessary bending down or over.
✳ Remember your posture. Keep your stomach in, your back straight, your shoulders back with your ears over your shoulders, and your chest up and out.
✳ Don't always hold baby on the same side. Swap over (this can be hard to remember if you're, say, right-handed and automatically put baby on your left hip), so one side doesn't become overburdened.
✳ Rest as much as possible. When you're tired, your posture gets weaker.

POSTNATAL YOGA

The first six weeks after the birth are known as the fourth and last stage of labour, and it is a very special time for you and for your baby. Try to take it easy, and get all the help you can from your loved ones. After this, you could slowly prepare your body with some gentle yoga poses to feel empowered both physically and emotionally. If you have had a C-section, it is recommended you wait for 12 weeks after birth, but always consult your doctor first. Danai is a pre- and postnatal yoga instructor at Bodyism and this is the sequence she recommends for all brand new mums.

'These simple postnatal yoga poses will help strengthen your abdomen, arms, legs and pelvic floor, increase your stamina and ease the stress of sleep loss. More important, you will feel centred, grounded and uplifted. Take the time to nourish and nurture yourself amid the new challenges in your life, so you can do the same for your baby!'
BY DANAI KOUGIOULI

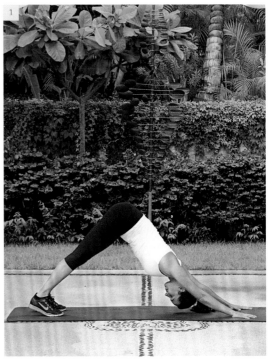

1. Downward-facing dog

Start by holding the pose for 5 breaths, gradually building to 10 breaths.

2. Plank to downward-facing dog

From downward-facing dog, move the shoulders over the wrists, bringing the body into plank position, focusing on tightening your abdomen, then lift the hips high back to downward-facing dog. Repeat 5 times.

3. Downward-facing dog - Kegel exercises (pelvic floor toning)

In downward-facing dog, lift your pelvic floor (quickly squeeze the muscles that stop the flow of urine), squeeze for 5 breaths, hold for 5 breaths, and release for 5 breaths, then repeat 5 times.

4. Warrior II

Build strength in your body by stretching the legs and ankles, groin, chest and lungs and shoulders. Hold for 5 breaths, then repeat on the other side.

5. Mountain pose, hands in prayer at the heart

As you bow your head to your heart, take a moment to honour your body, and be grateful for your baby!

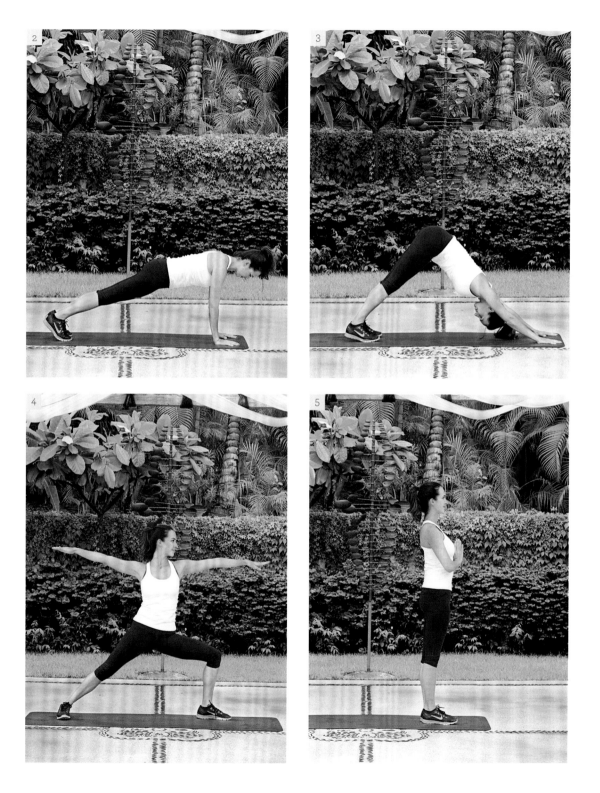

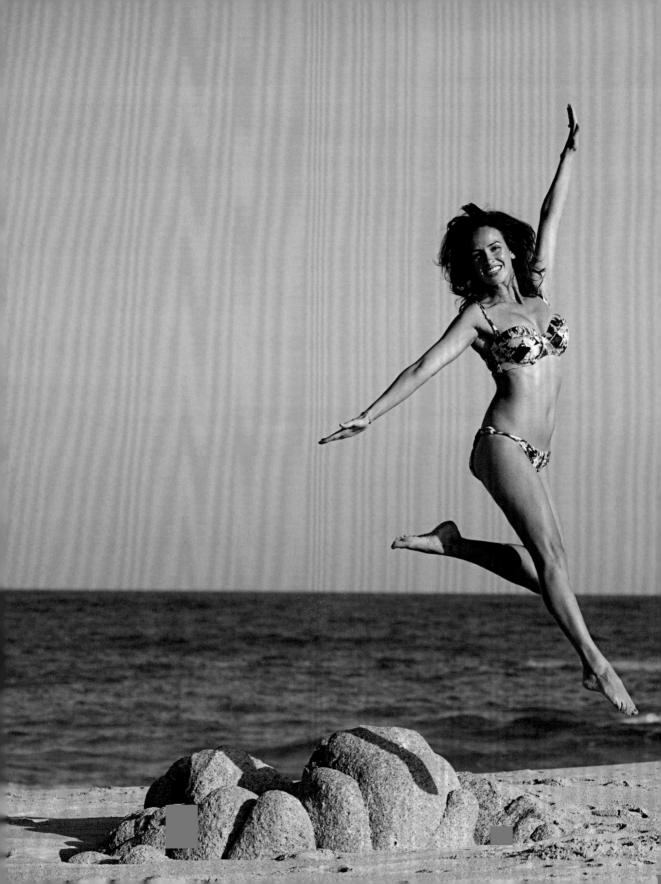

CHAPTER 7

HOW TO GET YOUR BODY BACK

GET-YOUR-BODY-BACK WORKOUT

This chapter is for all the mums out there who have never quite managed to get their bodies back after having children. I get a lot of female clients who had babies six months or even years ago, and they often ask me how to get rid of their 'mum tum' – the soft, jiggly, post-baby stomach. It can often include a fold of fat even when the rest of the body is fairly slim.

The good news is that, even if you had your baby several years ago, it's never too late. You may not restore your pre-baby stomach back to exactly how it was, but you can achieve something that resembles it with a few small changes to your life and an exercise routine.

Diet-wise, one of my first recommendations is to take a good-quality fish oil supplement. Studies show that this switches on the fat-burning hormones and – crucially – turns off the fat-storing ones. Fish oils also encourage your body to burn fat around your mid-section, which is often the area most women want to change after having children.

Secondly, if you haven't been doing them already, get into the habit of doing your pelvic-floor exercises every day. You should do these soon after giving birth. In fact, every woman should do them every day, whether she has had children or not. But even if you haven't done any, start now. Keeping your pelvic-floor muscles strong acts as an internal corset and pulls your stomach in from the inside (this isn't the technical term, but it's a simple way of describing what happens in general), creating a more toned and flat-looking mid-section. Your pelvic-floor muscles are the ones you would use if you were trying to stop yourself from peeing. Squeeze and clench them (as if you were stopping the flow) for a few seconds. Do 15–20 squeezes, five times a day. (The great thing about these exercises is you can do them anywhere at any time, and nobody will even know you're doing them.)

As well as pelvic-floor exercises, here are some other exercises that are great for targeting that 'mum tum'. Try to perform this workout 2–4 times a week on non-consecutive days but, if you haven't exercised for a while, build up to this slowly, with 2 workouts a week to begin with. When you find that you have more energy and are getting stronger, you can increase the amount of time you train. Remember to listen to your body and keep eating Clean & Lean.

EXERCISE	REPS	SETS	REST
Squat with push press	12–15	2–3	30 secs
Row with towel	10–15	2–3	30 secs
Squat	12–15	2–3	30 secs
Triceps dip	8–10	2–3	30 secs
Opposites	10/side	2–3	30 secs
T	12–15	2–3	60 secs

'I'M SLIMMER NOW THAN BEFORE I GOT PREGNANT'

'I'm such an advocate of Clean & Lean; it's done such amazing things for me. I gained nearly 4 stone during my pregnancy, but I now weigh a stone less than my pre-pregnancy weight, thanks to Clean & Lean.

'I had a C-section, so it took quite a while to recover, which meant really small amounts of exercise. My baby was also such a bad sleeper, and I felt exhausted all the time. I happened upon Clean & Lean completely by accident. On a rare evening relaxing in the bath I was reading a magazine featuring James helping a new mum who felt tired. Initially, I started the diet to give myself energy, but the weight dropped off as an added benefit. It took a year, but by the time I went back to work I'd lost everything I'd gained and more. I felt totally revitalised. I've encouraged others to become Clean & Lean and they've had similar results. My husband lost over 17lb just by having the same meals as me. My son is now two and a half and I still follow the principles, occasionally getting the book out to refresh my memory. Foolishly, I'd always thought it was better to eat sugar than fat – how wrong I was! This diet is amazing.'

by Olivia Herbert

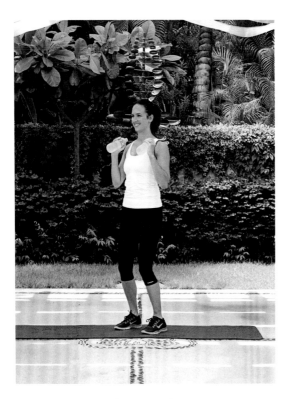

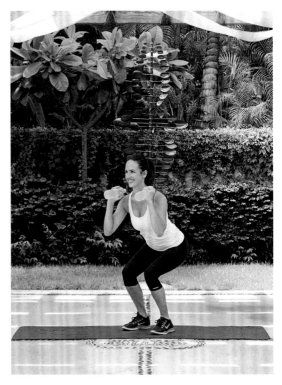

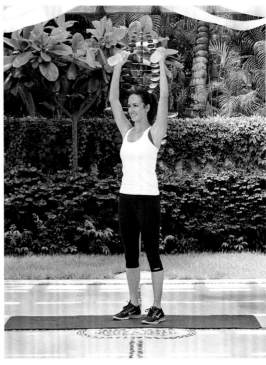

Squat with push press

Start position: Stand with your hips shoulder-width apart and holding a weight, or even a large bottle of water, in each hand. Squat down, keeping your chest open, and raise your hands in front of your shoulders. Engage your core by pulling your belly button in towards the spine.

The movement: Stand up by pushing through the heels and bring the hips forwards so that the knees and hips are extended. As the hips fully extend, push the water bottles (or weights) over your head so that the arms, hips and knees are fully extended. Then slowly lower the water bottles (or weights) to the starting position and repeat 12–15 times.

*top tip
This exercise will help strengthen your glutes and shoulders.

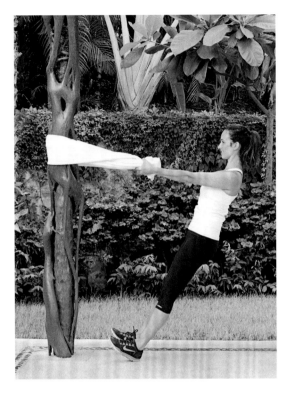

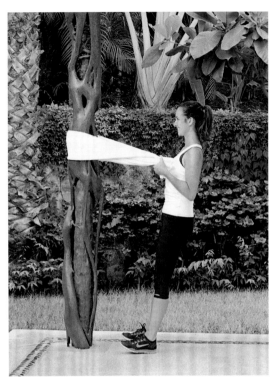

Row with towel

Start position: Wrap a towel securely around a post or narrow tree trunk. Stand near the post or tree and take the ends of the towel in your hands, then extend your arms out fully, leaning backwards. Keep the weight on your heels and a straight line from the top of your head to your heels. Engage your core by pulling your belly button in towards the spine.

The movement: Keeping your elbows tucked in, pull your body up so your hands are brought close to your chest whilst your body remains in a straight line. Return to the start position and repeat 10–15 times.

*top tip

This exercise will strengthen your back muscles, which are essential for improving your posture – a key area for a new mother carrying her baby. It is a great exercise to do outdoors.

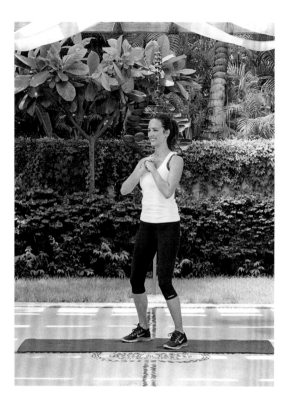
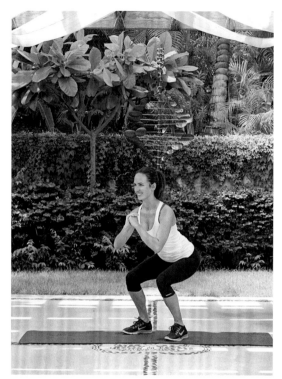

Squat

Start position: Stand with your feet hip-width apart and hands clenched in front of your chest. Engage your core by pulling your belly button in towards the spine.

The movement: Keeping your hands clenched in front of your chest, squat down by pushing your hips back and bending the knees until your thighs are parallel to the floor. Throughout the movement, keep your torso upright. Return to the start position by pushing through the hips and the heels and repeat 12–15 times.

*top tip
This exercise will help strengthen your glutes, hamstrings and thighs.

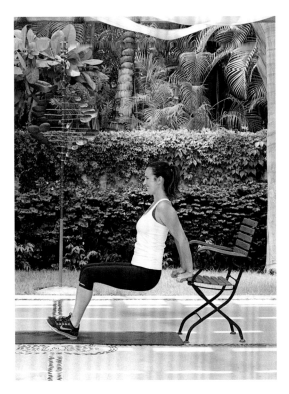
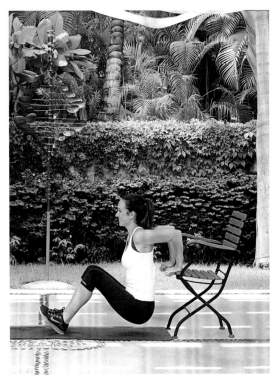

Triceps dip

Start position: Using a step/low chair/bench, sit your back and butt against the front and place your hands behind you on the edge. Keep your knees at 90 degrees, heels on the floor and toes up in the air. Lift your body up so that your hips are off the step and level with your hands. Engage your core by pulling your belly button in towards the spine.

The movement: Slowly lower yourself down towards the ground by bending the arms until your elbows are at 90 degrees. Then return to the start position by pushing your palms down on the support. Repeat 8–10 times.

*top tip

This exercise will strengthen your tricep muscles and help fight off any 'bingo wings'.

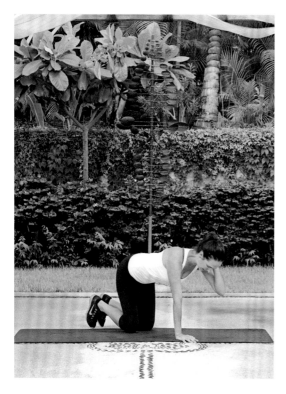
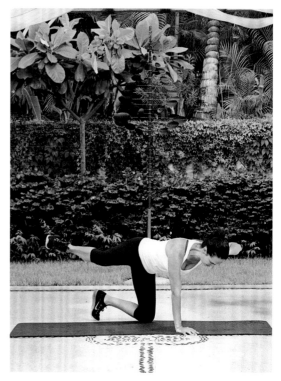

Opposites

Start position: Support yourself on your hands and knees with hands under shoulders and knees under hips. Maintain a flat back and keep your neck in a straight line with your back. Place your left hand on the base of your neck. Engage your core by pulling your belly button in towards the spine.

The movement: Lift your right leg up as if showing the outside of your thigh to the sky, keeping the knee bent, whilst you simultaneously raise your left elbow to the sky. Finish so that your right knee and your left elbow are level with your back. Aim to keep your hips and shoulders parallel to the floor throughout the movement. Slowly return to the start position. Repeat 10 times on each side.

*top tip

This is an incredibly effective exercise to help improve the strength of your postural muscles and lower back.

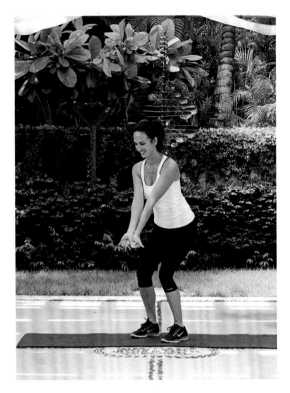

T

Start position: Stand with your feet hip-width apart. Bend your knees and lean forwards so your torso is at a 45-degree angle. Keep your head and back all in a straight line, your shoulders back and down and your hands directly below your chest with fists clenched and thumbs pointing outward. Engage your core by pulling your belly button in towards the spine.

The movement: Keeping your body still and your core engaged, raise your arms out to the sides to form a 'T' shape, then return to the start position. Repeat 12–15 times.

BREATHE YOURSELF SLIMMER

This is a great breathing exercise to strengthen your lower abdominal muscles – it will help to pull in that little pouch stomach many women have under their belly button. The move will also keep your back strong and healthy:

✳ Start on all fours with your back straight and your arms slightly bent at the elbows. Your ears should be in line with your shoulders and hips.

✳ Relax your abdominals and take a big breath from the belly, so it expands towards the floor.

✳ Slowly exhale and draw your belly button towards your spine, simultaneously doing a pelvic-floor exercise (see p. 150). Your back should remain straight at all times.

✳ Once the air is completely gone, hold the belly towards the spine for 5 seconds.

✳ Repeat the process 20 times.

HOW OUR COVER GIRL GOT HER BODY BACK

'After I had Charlotte, I worried that my body – and fitness – had regressed and that I'd never get them back. My ribcage and hips felt wider, so my tops and jeans looked and felt tight, even when I started to lose weight. But that's completely normal – they widen in pregnancy to make room for your growing baby and shrink back to their normal size within a year of giving birth.

'My biggest tip is to start slowly. When I began exercising again, I started off doing one or two hip extensions at a time, then I slowly built it up. Alongside these moves, I walked every day and did pelvic-floor exercises. I kept an eye on my posture because good posture makes you look slimmer and strengthens your core, which helps your stomach muscles fuse back together. I didn't need to lift weights because I was lifting an ever-growing Charlotte all the time – she did wonders for toning my arms!

'I also recommend wearing a corset after you have children. Ideally, you should start wearing it around six weeks after you give birth – a bit longer if you've had a C-section, and only if you're recovering well. Wearing it for a few hours a day pulls the stomach muscles (which come apart during pregnancy) back together, making your tummy look flatter and more toned. I had to build up to it. I managed an hour a day in the early months, and then gradually increased the amount. I didn't always remember to put it on, but it definitely helped tighten my tummy back up.

'I tried to have only Clean & Lean foods in the house so I wasn't tempted by sugar when I was sleep-deprived. I kept my energy levels up with lots of little healthy snacks. I often slow-cooked meat with plenty of vegetables because it was an easy dish to prepare that cooked itself and didn't involve lots of fiddly preparation. This way, I had something in the fridge when I needed a quick meal. Most mornings I blended anything green we had in the house (like broccoli, peppers, kale, spinach, etc.) with a squeeze of fresh lemon juice, some ginger and Himalayan sea salt and kick-started my day with a lovely green juice. This definitely helped pick me up when I'd been up in the night with Charlotte. And it takes the same amount of time to prepare as a coffee – just throw everything in a blender and you're there!

'I didn't deprive myself and I didn't cut out any food groups – I just ate Clean & Lean and listened to my body, and by about nine months it was back to how it was pre-pregnancy. I'm glad I took my time. Because I was eating well I felt better, I slept better and my milk supply was good for Charlotte. And when weight comes off slowly and steadily, it stays off for longer. So don't rush to lose your mummy tummy. Just take it slowly, give yourself a break and never feel bad about the fact your body isn't back to how it was. You've created a new little person and nurtured them – you're fantastic and never forget it.'

*top tip

Use your juicer or smoothie-maker frequently for a quick and healthy boost. It's the fastest way to give your body nutrients when you are tired or have limited time!

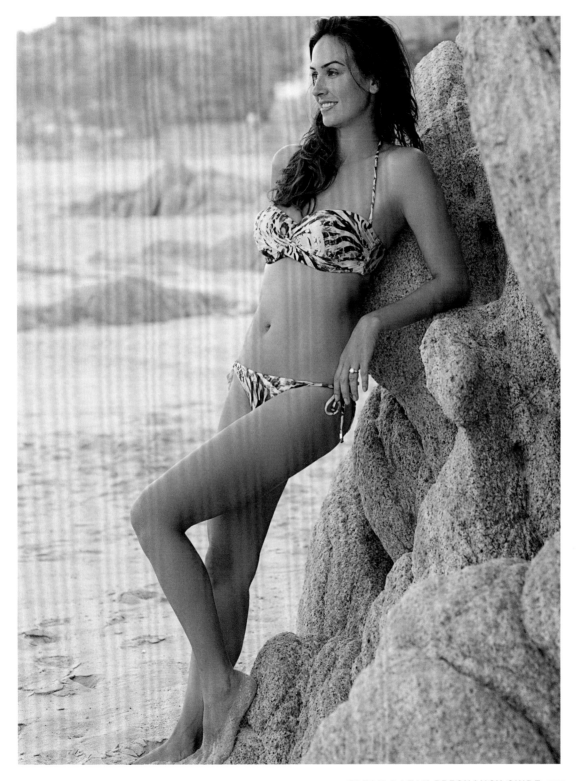

'I'M SURPRISED HOW MUCH WEIGHT I'VE LOST'

'After the birth of my son in October 2011, getting back into shape wasn't a huge concern for me. I just wanted to enjoy the precious moments of becoming a new parent. However, after a while I had a sort of mid-life crisis and decided I wanted to become fit and healthy. I was talking to a friend about it and she shared her secret – the Clean & Lean Diet and the cookbook. I got the books, started buying organic meat, fruit and vegetables from the weekend farmers' markets and cutting out sugar and preservatives. The books were so easy to follow and I realised it wasn't really a diet; it was a way of life. And I just saw the weight drop off.

'I've always been into exercising, but not regularly. In the past I went on exercise binges where I'd work out regularly, then I'd get bored or lose motivation and give up altogether. But I followed the simple moves in the book and loved them. Within a few days, I had more energy and felt so positive that I actually wanted to go for a run! Before I had had to drag myself to the gym.

'The last time I weighed myself I was surprised at how much weight I've lost since becoming Clean & Lean and how easily it has come off. My family and friends have started commenting on how good I look and that has kept me going as well. When I'm asked what my secret is, I tell people: "Clean & Lean".

'I'm pregnant again and, although this pregnancy is so different from the first, I still remain focused and try to avoid sugar, buy organic and I still pull out the cookbook regularly to keep me on track. I'm a firm believer that looking and feeling your best is 90 per cent diet and 10 per cent exercise – plus a fair bit of positive thinking. The journey to losing my pregnancy weight the first time was so straightforward and enjoyable, I'm looking forward to doing it again.'

by Heather Budiselik

SLEEP YOURSELF SLIMMER

When I speak to new mums who want to get in shape, one of the biggest obstacles they face is the fact they feel so tired all the time. Being a mum is the most rewarding job in the world, but it's also the most relentless and tiring. Whether you're a stay-at-home mum, a part-time mum or a mum who works full-time, there's no break. When you're not being a mum, you're working. Even when you're not with your baby, you're thinking about them. It can be tough physically too – especially in the early days – and emotionally as you worry endlessly about them being well fed, well rested and happy. There are no weekends off, no lunch breaks, no holidays and no sick pay! And I've yet to see a baby congratulate a mum on a job well done!

A really important part of getting your body back is to have plenty of rest so you feel recharged. Even a minute of meditation can achieve this, and I'm going to show you how. Getting enough sleep impacts hugely on our appetites and the foods we choose. After a good night's sleep, or even some meditation, you will naturally and happily choose Clean & Lean food that work for your body, making you look better and, more importantly, feel better, whereas after little or broken sleep you'll crave sugar, processed carbs and caffeine. This is because these foods briefly cause energy levels to rise, by creating a huge spike in our blood-sugar levels; but this spike is followed by a crash – which is why you feel groggy after eating a whole bag of sugary snacks. You literally have a sugar hangover! You then get sucked into a cycle of tiredness and sugar cravings – you eat sugar because you're always tired, but you're always tired because you eat sugar. You don't feel that way after eating a bowl of fresh berries, though – they will give you a strong, sustained energy boost to help you be a better mama. So think long term – choose foods that make you feel good for a long time.

HOW TO CREATE LONG-LASTING ENERGY

✳ Lay off the coffee. A couple of coffees, teas or green teas to get you going in the morning are fine. I do it myself. But don't have any after midday – even if you've been up all night with your baby. Coffee after lunch will still be in your system at bedtime, so you won't fall into the type of lovely, restorative sleep you need to keep your metabolism – and health – in tip-top condition. Most of us get a 4pm energy slump, but work through it with fresh air and Clean & Lean snacks, and if you really feel you need something, have a green tea. Move around a bit and drink plenty of water.
✳ Avoid alcohol. Lots of mums have a glass of wine after the kids' bedtime to help them unwind, but it doesn't work. Alcohol is incredibly stressful on your body (as well as being full of sugar, it can dehydrate you and you tend to wake up earlier the morning after you've been drinking).
✳ Eat more nuts, beans, turkey, fish and eggs. They're rich in tryptophan and studies show that eating this in the day helps your sleep better at night. Remember, better sleep = a better body and a better mama.

Avoid sugar. It's a stimulant that will keep you awake. So stay away from the following after lunchtime:
✳ White refined sugar
✳ Fruit juices and energy drinks
✳ White, non-organic pasta, bread and rice
✳ Alcohol (see above)
✳ Cakes, sweets, biscuits and ice cream
✳ Low-fat foods, such as diet yogurts, most processed breakfast cereals, 'health' bars and muffins
✳ Anything that contains an ingredient ending in 'ose' (sucrose, glucose, maltose, lactose, dextrose and fructose); it's basically another word for sugar
✳ Anything containing high-fructose corn syrup; again, it's sugar by another name
✳ All sweeteners

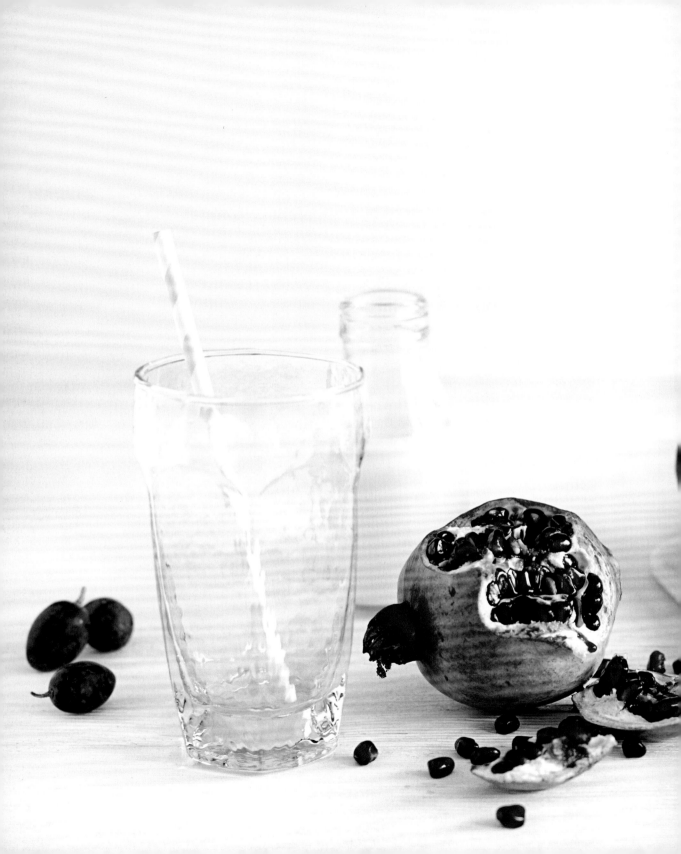

CHAPTER 8

QUICK CLEAN & LEAN RECIPES

THE RECIPES

Like the rest of this book, these recipes are for women who are either trying to get pregnant, who are pregnant or who are new mums. You can enjoy them in all three of your trimesters and I've deliberately kept them as simple and quick as possible. Feel free to tweak them or substitute ingredients you don't like for Clean & Lean foods you do like.

*it's easy
Vary this omelette with toppings of your choice – broccoli, spinach, goat's cheese, etc.

*top tip
Eggs are a fantastic source of quality protein, which is essential in pregnancy. They're also full of B vitamins that convert food into energy.

Tomato, Rocket and Mushroom Omelette
Serves 1

Ingredients
2 eggs
freshly ground black pepper
4–5 cherry tomatoes, halved
5–6 button mushrooms, thinly sliced
a handful of rocket

Method

1 Beat the eggs and some ground black pepper in a bowl.

2 Place a non-stick pan over a medium heat, then pour in the egg mixture and swirl to coat the pan evenly. Allow the base of the omelette to firm slightly, then top with the tomatoes and mushrooms and cook to warm through.

3 When the omelette is cooked to your liking (make sure the egg is well done when you're pregnant), remove it from the heat and scatter over the rocket. Serve immediately.

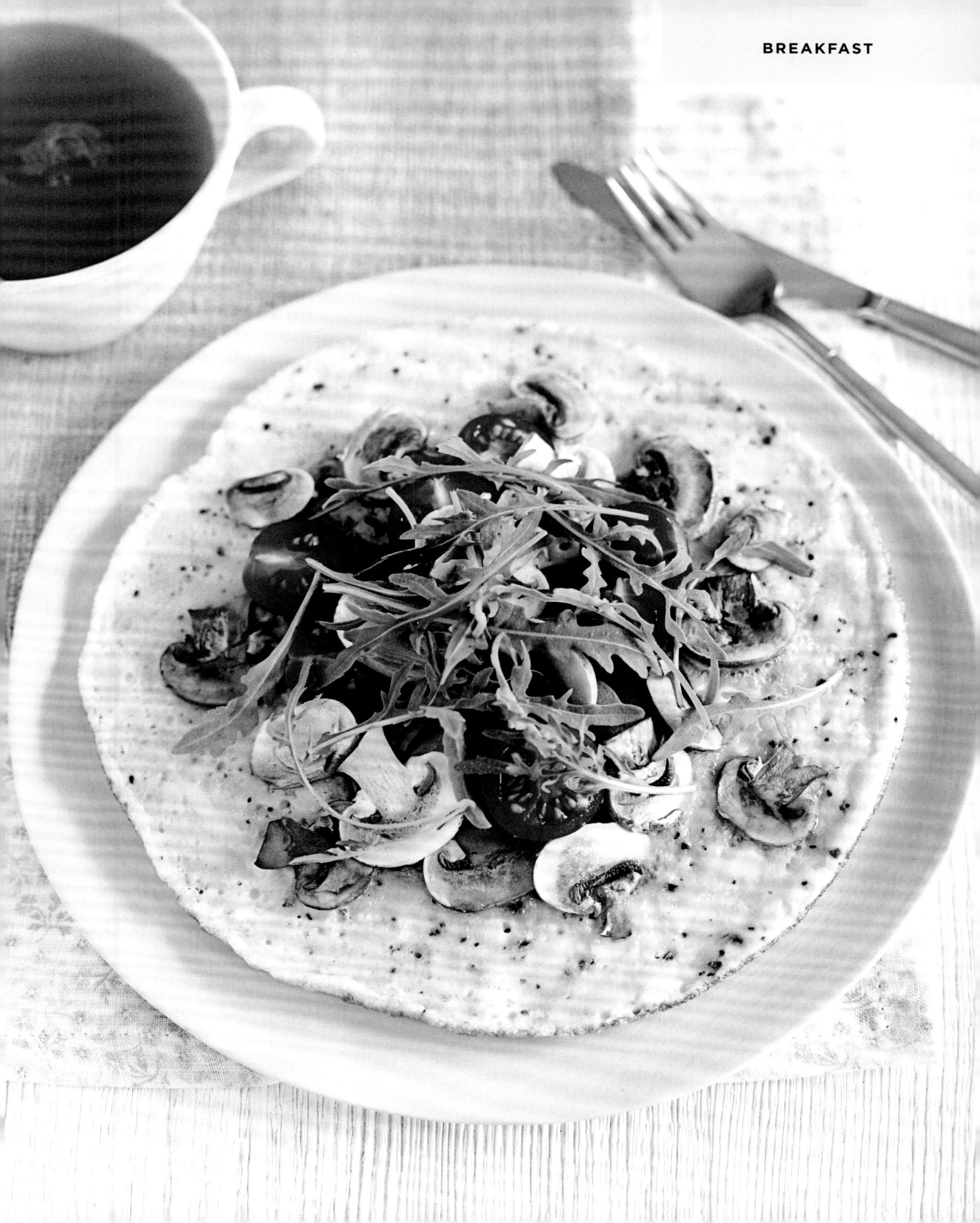

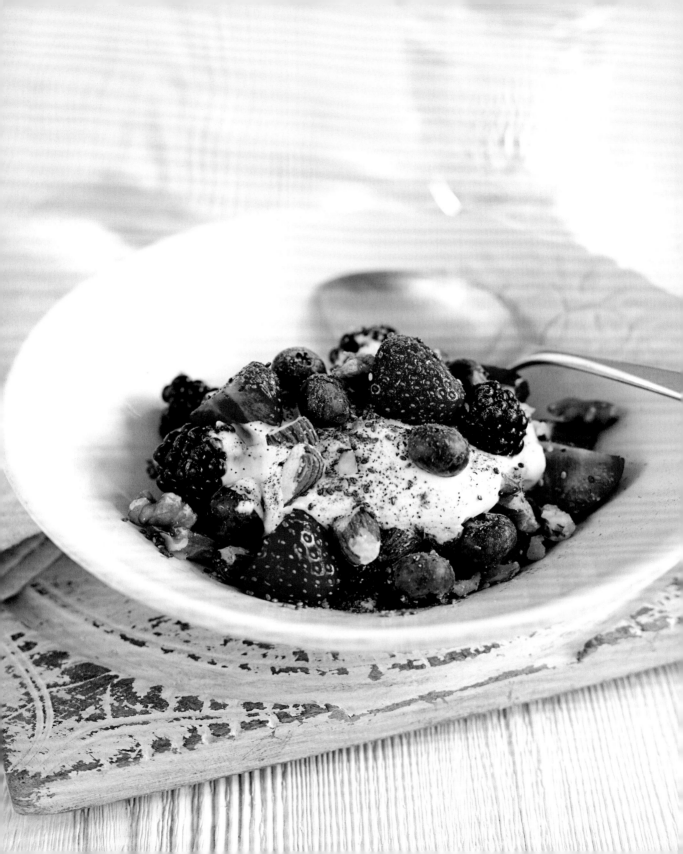

Nut and Berry Breakfast

Serves 2

Ingredients

a small handful of walnuts
a small handful of almonds
a good sprinkling of chia seeds
3 good handfuls of your favourite berries
   (try blueberries, blackberries, raspberries,
   strawberries, etc.)
4 tablespoons organic full-fat Greek yogurt
1 teaspoon ground cinnamon

Method

1 Place all the nuts and seeds into a food-processor, and pulse until they are coarsely chopped.

2 Place a layer of berries in the bottom of a bowl, then add a layer of the nut mix and top with a layer of organic yogurt. Repeat this layering, finishing with some berries and a sprinkling of cinnamon.

*top tip

Blend up your favourite fruits and vegetables with plenty of ice. It will satisfy your craving for something cold and sweet, plus deliver a hit of nutrients to you and your baby.

Clean & Lean Oat Pancakes

Serves 2–4

Ingredients

100g rolled oats
200g full-fat cottage cheese or ricotta
4 eggs
1 teaspoon ground cinnamon
manuka honey
Greek yogurt

Method

1 Blend the rolled oats, cottage cheese or ricotta, eggs and cinnamon in a food-processor.

2 Pour a ladleful of the mixture into a non-stick frying pan placed over a medium heat and cook for 2–3 minutes on each side.

3 Remove the pancake from the pan and keep it warm while you cook the remaining mixture in the same way.

4 Serve the pancakes with a drizzle of manuka honey and a spoonful of Greek yogurt.

*top tip

Greek yogurt is packed with calcium, so is a great go-to food for pregnancy and breastfeeding. It's perfect with fruit and muesli for breakfast and also makes a delicious mid-morning snack.

Baked Eggs with Tomatoes, Spinach and Goat's Cheese

Serves 2

Ingredients

50g spinach
2 teaspoons olive oil
2 handfuls of cherry tomatoes, halved
1 large garlic clove, finely chopped
75g goat's cheese
2 eggs
freshly ground black pepper

Method

1 Preheat the oven to 180°C/gas mark 4.

2 Place the spinach in a colander and pour over boiling water to cover and wilt. Leave to cool, then gently squeeze out any excess water.

3 Mix together the olive oil, tomatoes, spinach and garlic and divide between 2 small ovenproof dishes. Crumble the goat's cheese over the vegetables and, without breaking the yolk, crack an egg over the top of each and season with black pepper. Bake in the oven for 10–15 minutes, ensuring the yolk is cooked through as this is important during pregnancy. Serve hot.

*top tip

Ginger tea is good for reducing morning sickness. Nettle tea contains magnesium, calcium and iron, all of which are good for energy. And peppermint tea is great for helping your digestion, which often slows down during pregnancy.

Nutty Granola

Serves 2

Ingredients

50g dried prunes, roughly chopped
60g jumbo rolled oats
4 tablespoons honey
40g chopped mixed Brazil nuts and almonds

Method

1 Preheat the oven to 150°C/gas mark 2.

2 Mix all the ingredients together. Spread the mixture on to a baking tray and bake in the oven for 10–15 minutes.

3 Turn the oven temperature down to 110°C/gas mark ¼ and bake for a further 30 minutes. Remove from the oven and leave to cool completely before serving.

*top tip

If you don't have any time to make breakfast, just grab half an avocado, slice it up and have it on a few oatcakes.

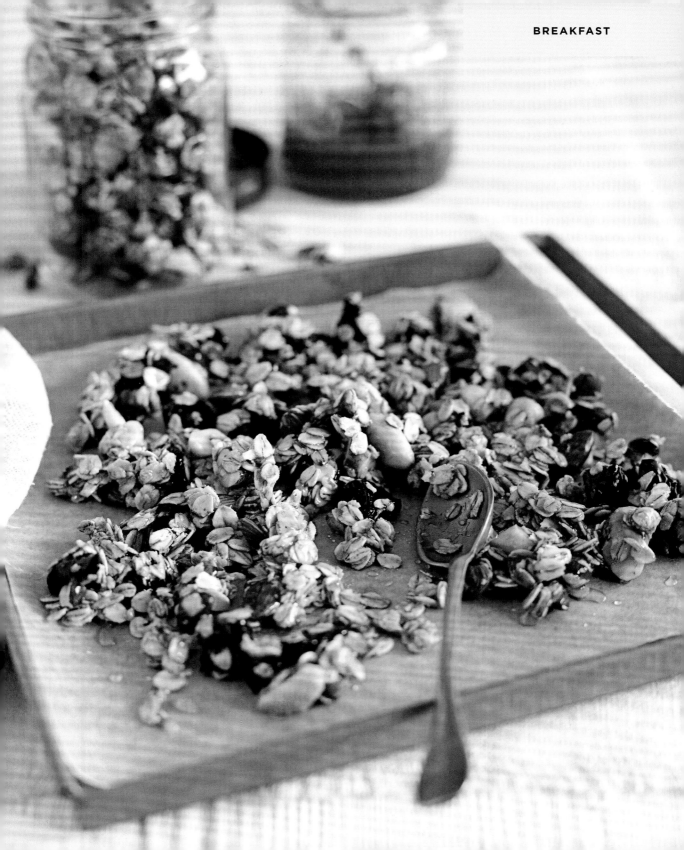

Fruit Skewers and Honey
Serves 2

Ingredients
4 strawberries, washed
8 blackberries, washed
½ mango, peeled and chopped into bite-sized chunks
2 kiwis, peeled and chopped into bite-sized chunks
2 tablespoons manuka honey
1 teaspoon ground cinnamon

Method

1 Preheat the oven to 150°C/gas mark 2.

2 You will need 4 skewers. If you are using wooden ones, soak them in water for at least 30 minutes beforehand.

3 Thread 2 pieces of each fruit on to each skewer.

4 In a bowl, mix the manuka honey with the cinnamon. Using a pastry brush, glaze the fruit skewers with the honey mixture.

5 Place the skewers on a baking tray and cook in the oven for about 5 minutes, turning every minute or so, until the fruit is soft and lightly charred. Serve immediately.

*top tip
Fresh fruit is packed with nutrients and full of fibre, and it is extremely important that you eat lots during your pregnancy. These skewers make it easy and are simply delicious.

Scrambled Eggs and Smoked Salmon
Serves 2

Ingredients
4 eggs
freshly ground black pepper
100g smoked salmon
chopped herbs (such as dill or basil), to garnish

Method

1 Beat the eggs in a bowl with some black pepper.

2 Place a non-stick saucepan on a low heat, pour the eggs into the pan and cook, whisking gently, until they are cooked through.

3 Transfer the eggs to serving plates, add the smoked salmon and garnish with chopped herbs. Serve immediately.

*top tip
Smoked salmon is an excellent pregnancy food – high in omega-3 fatty acids, plus it makes a simple, quick breakfast, lunch or snack, with eggs, in a salad or on a slice of rye bread.

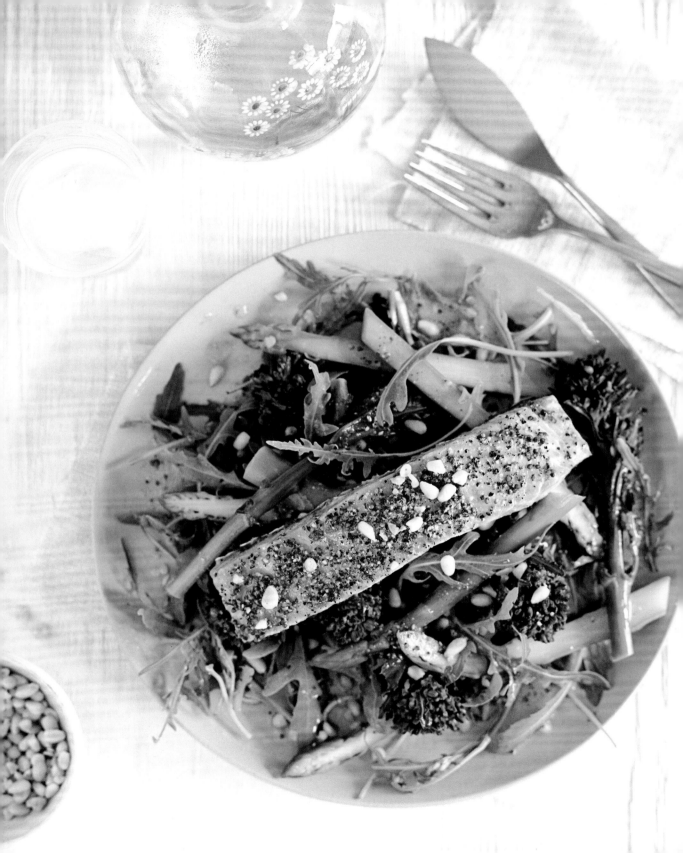

Salmon and Vegetable Medley

Serves 2

Ingredients

1 teaspoon wholegrain mustard
juice of 1 lemon
freshly ground black pepper
2 salmon fillets
350g asparagus
250g broccoli, broken into florets
100g rocket
1 tablespoon chopped pine nuts

Method

1 Preheat the oven to 200°C/gas mark 6.

2 Mix the mustard, lemon juice and some black pepper together to make a marinade. Rub the salmon with a little of the mixture, then place in the oven and cook for 10 minutes.

3 Meanwhile, steam the asparagus and broccoli for 15 minutes, or until soft.

4 Divide the rocket between 2 plates and top with the asparagus and broccoli. Place a salmon fillet on each plate and pour the remaining marinade over the top. Sprinkle with the chopped pine nuts and serve.

Ginger and Sweet Potato Soup

Serves 4

Ingredients

1 tablespoon sesame oil
1 small onion, diced
2 celery sticks, chopped
5cm piece of fresh ginger, peeled and finely chopped
2 garlic cloves, finely chopped
1 litre organic vegetable stock
3–4 sweet potatoes, peeled and chopped into
    evenly sized chunks
freshly ground black pepper
chopped fresh coriander, to serve

Method

1 Heat the oil in a large saucepan over a medium heat. Add the onion, celery, ginger and garlic and sauté for a few minutes until softened, but not coloured.

2 Stir in the stock and sweet potatoes and season with black pepper. Bring to a simmer and cook for 15–20 minutes, until the sweet potatoes are tender.

3 Remove from the heat and leave to cool slightly, then blend the soup until smooth. Add more water if you prefer a thinner soup.

4 Return the soup to the pan and warm through. Taste and add more black pepper if necessary, before serving scattered with coriander.

*top tip

Ginger is great for soothing nausea and this soup is easy to prepare. It can be made in bulk and frozen so you can have some on standby.

Butternut Squash and Lentil Salad

Serves 2

Ingredients

1 garlic clove, crushed
2 teaspoons thyme leaves
1 tablespoon olive oil
450g butternut squash, peeled and cut
  into evenly sized chunks
½ onion, thinly sliced
400g cooked puy lentils
80g spinach
25g flat-leaf parsley, finely chopped
juice of 1 lemon
freshly ground black pepper

Method

1 Preheat the oven to 200°C/gas mark 6.

2 Mix the garlic, thyme and olive oil together and brush over the butternut squash. Place in a roasting tray with the onion and roast in the oven for 25 minutes, until slightly caramelised.

3 Toss the puy lentils with the spinach and divide between 2 plates. Add the butternut squash, scatter over the parsley and sprinkle with the lemon juice. Season with black pepper and serve immediately.

Prawn, Avocado and Grapefruit salad

Serves 2

Ingredients

1 large pink grapefruit
2 tablespoons extra virgin olive oil
a large handful of rocket
150g cooked, shelled prawns
1 avocado, peeled, stoned and chopped
2 rye crackers or 4 oatcakes, to serve

Method

1 Peel the grapefruit, removing all the white pith. Chop the flesh into chunks and reserve any juice in a bowl. Add the olive oil to the grapefruit juice.

2 Divide the rocket between 2 plates, then top with the grapefruit chunks. Drizzle the grapefruit juice and olive oil over the salad, toss gently and top with the prawns and avocado. Serve with the rye crackers or oatcakes.

*top tip

Lentils, like many beans and pulses, are nutrient-rich and a good source of iron, folate and zinc. Plus they're full of fibre – especially important for keeping your digestive system, which can be disrupted by pregnancy, in good working order.

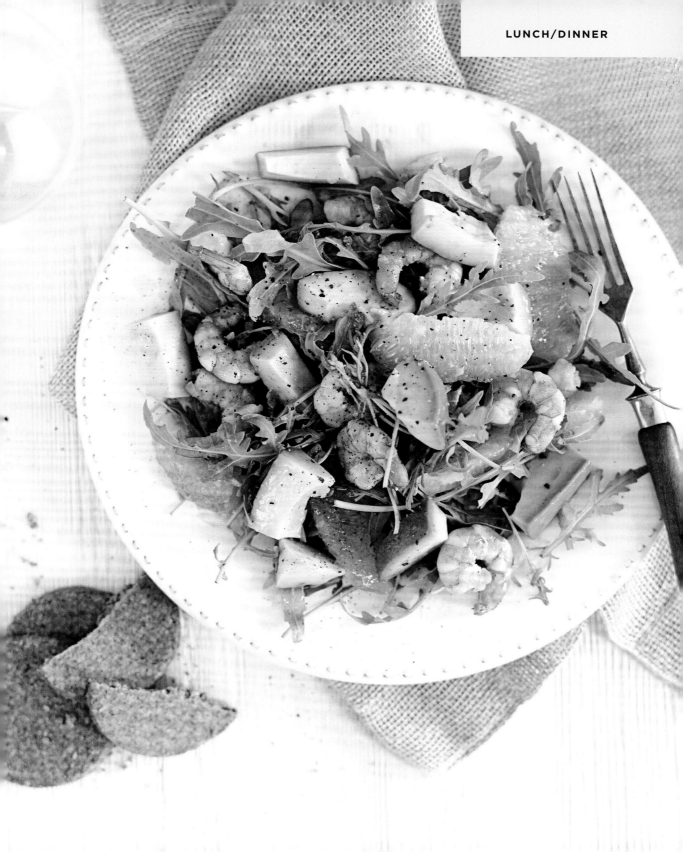

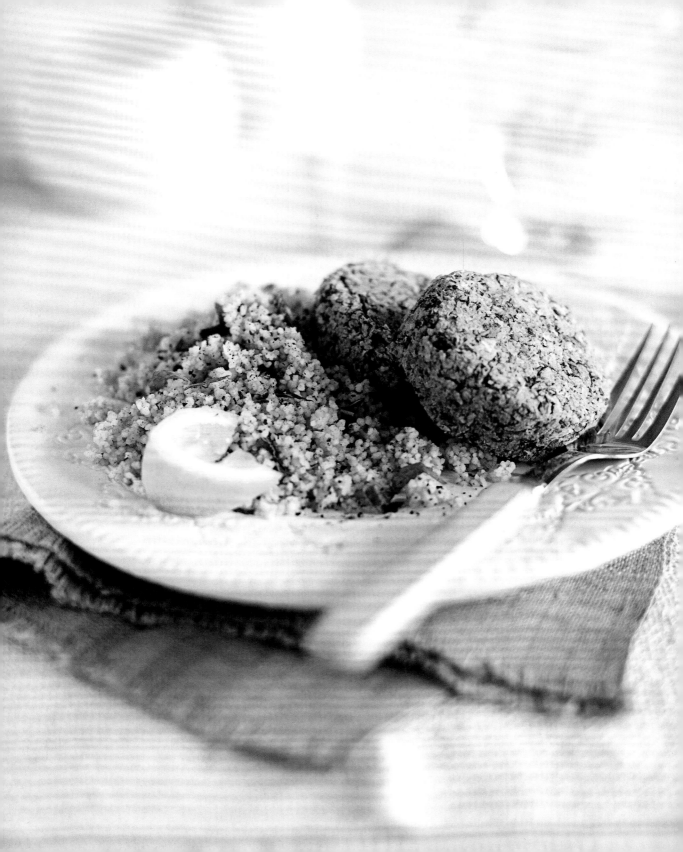

Lemon and Coriander Chickpea Burgers

Serves 2

Ingredients
1 tablespoon olive oil
1 garlic clove, crushed
1 teaspoon ground coriander
250g cooked chickpeas
80g curly kale
100g couscous
juice of 1 lemon, plus lemon wedges to serve
15g fresh mint, finely chopped
1 teaspoon ground turmeric

Method

1 Preheat the oven to 200°C/gas mark 6.

2 Place the olive oil in a frying pan over a medium heat. Add the crushed garlic and coriander and stir for 2–3 minutes. Remove from the heat and place in a bowl.

3 Blend the chickpeas and kale in a food-processor, add to the bowl with the garlic and coriander and mix well.

4 Divide the chickpea mixture into 4 burgers, arrange on a baking sheet and cook in the oven for 15–20 minutes.

5 Meanwhile, make the couscous according to the packet instructions, then gently stir through the lemon juice, chopped mint and turmeric.

6 Serve the chickpea burgers with the couscous and lemon wedges for squeezing.

Mackerel with Toasted Rye

Serves 1

Ingredients
1 cooked mackerel fillet
a pinch of smoked paprika
50g cottage cheese
juice of ½ orange
1 slice of rye bread
freshly ground black pepper

Method

1 In a bowl, divide the mackerel fillet into small pieces and sprinkle over the paprika. Mix together with the cottage cheese and orange juice.

2 Toast the rye bread and then spread with the mackerel mixture. Finish with a grind or two of black pepper and serve immediately.

*top tip

Eating oily fish twice a week during pregnancy has many benefits, both for mother and baby – it is a useful source of protein and good fats that are crucial components for the development of brain cells.

Herby Roast Chicken

Serves 4–6

Ingredients
1.6kg free-range chicken
2 sweet potatoes, peeled and sliced
4 carrots, peeled and sliced
2 yellow peppers, sliced
2 red onions, sliced
1 garlic bulb, broken into cloves
a small bunch of rosemary, thyme or sage, or a mixture
2 tablespoons olive oil
freshly ground black pepper
1 lemon
a drizzle of balsamic vinegar

Method

1 Preheat the oven to 240°C/gas mark 9 and take the chicken out of the fridge.

2 Place all the vegetables, the garlic and half the herbs in a large roasting tray and drizzle with 1 tablespoon of the olive oil. Season with black pepper and toss to combine.

3 Place the chicken in a separate roasting tray, season with pepper and drizzle with the remaining olive oil, rubbing it all over the bird.

4 With a sharp knife, prick the lemon all over and place inside the chicken's cavity with the remaining herbs.

5 Place both roasting trays in the oven and turn the heat down immediately to 200°C/gas mark 6. Cook for 1 hour 20 minutes.

6 Baste the chicken halfway through with the cooking juices and, if the vegetables look dry, add a splash of water to the tray to stop them burning. When the chicken is cooked, transfer it to a board to rest for 15 minutes or so.

7 Drizzle the roasted vegetables with a little balsamic vinegar and serve the chicken on top.

Garlic Chicken Stir-fry

Serves 2

Ingredients
1 teaspoon olive oil
2 skinless free-range chicken breasts, thinly sliced
5–6 broccoli florets
1 garlic clove, finely chopped
1 red chilli, finely chopped
2 red peppers, thinly sliced
1 tablespoon sesame seeds

Method

1 Heat the oil in a wok and stir-fry the chicken and broccoli for 5–10 minutes.

2 Add the garlic, chilli and red peppers and cook for a further minute.

3 Sprinkle with sesame seeds and serve immediately.

*top tip

Broccoli truly deserves to be classified a 'superfood' – loaded with vitamins and minerals, including vitamins A, C and K, as well as the all-important folate.

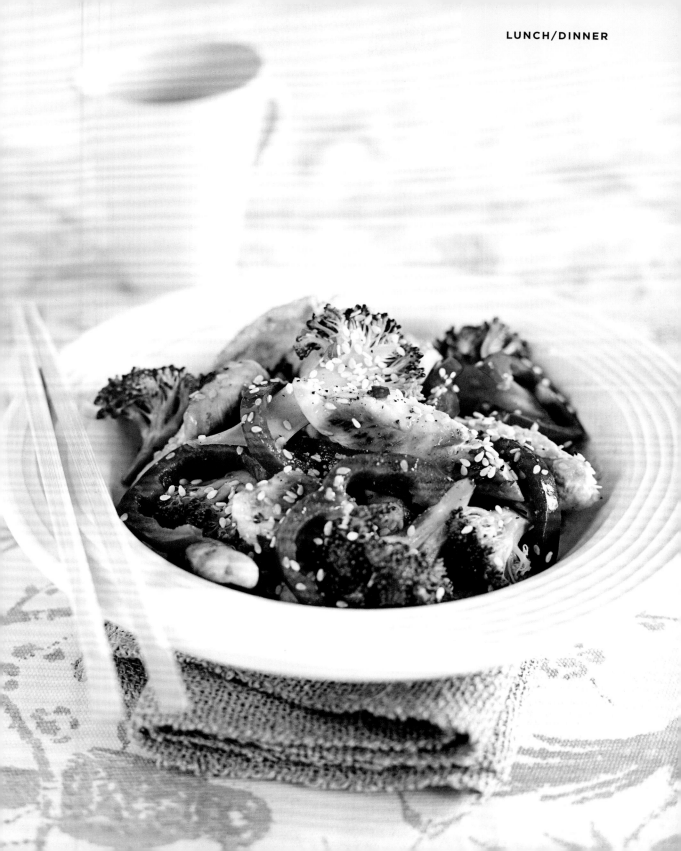

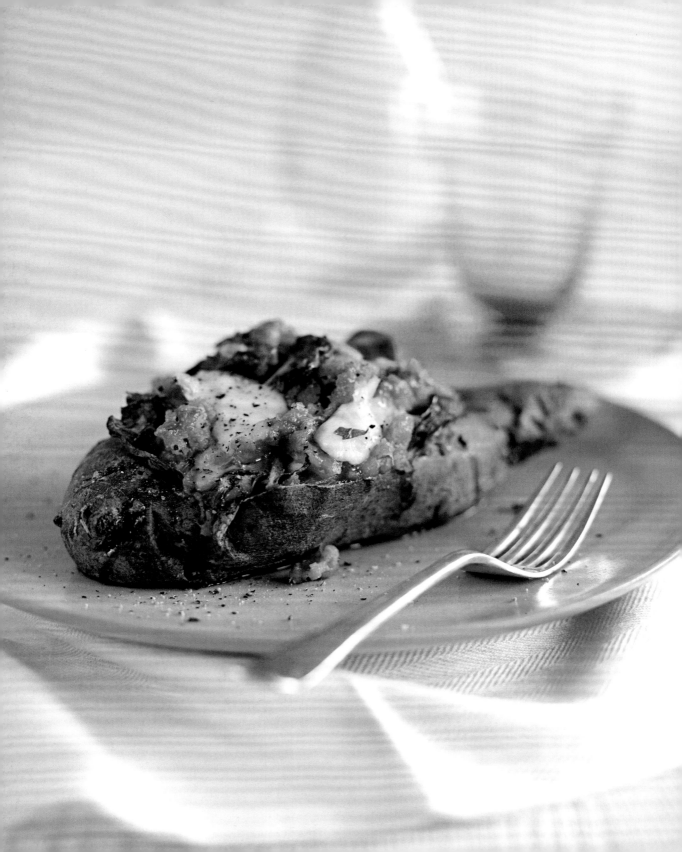

*top tip

Spinach is a great source of vitamin C, folate and fibre and a great food to have on hand throughout your pregnancy.

Baked Sweet Potato with Spinach and Mozzarella

Serves 2

Ingredients

2 large sweet potatoes
100g baby spinach
150g mozzarella cheese, diced
1 tablespoon olive oil
freshly ground black pepper

Method

1 Preheat the oven to 200°C/gas mark 6.

2 Prick the skins of the sweet potatoes and bake in the oven for 40 minutes, or until soft. Leave to cool.

3 Once the potatoes are cool, cut off the tops, scoop out the flesh and put in a bowl. Add the spinach, mozzarella and olive oil, and mix well. Season with ground black pepper.

4 Refill the potato skins with the mixture and return to the oven for a further 10 minutes to heat through.

Grilled Turkey and Rocket Wraps

Serves 2

Ingredients

4 large romaine lettuce leaves
50g cream cheese
a large handful of rocket
2 free-range turkey breasts, grilled and sliced
4 slices of fresh tomato
freshly ground black pepper

Method

1 Lay the lettuce leaves flat and spread a layer of cream cheese over each.

2 Add the rocket and top with the turkey. Add a slice of tomato to each 'wrap' and season with black pepper. Roll up the lettuce leaves and serve.

*top tip

Instead of eating white bread (a common pregnancy craving), have some wholegrain, wholewheat or quinoa bread instead, spread with organic nut butter.

Lamb and Apricot Tagine

Serves 4–6

Ingredients

1½ tablespoons olive oil

500g lean lamb, diced

1 large onion, roughly chopped

2 garlic cloves, finely chopped

1 tablespoon ras el hanout spice mix

1 teaspoon ground cumin

½ teaspoon ground ginger

1 cinnamon stick

400g tinned tomatoes

200g dried apricots

600ml chicken or vegetable stock

freshly ground black pepper

To serve

cooked quinoa

a handful of coriander

50 toasted almonds

Method

1 Preheat the oven to 180°C/gas mark 4.

2 Heat the olive oil in a flameproof casserole and brown the lamb on all sides. Transfer to a plate and add the onion to the pan, cooking for 3–4 mins until softened.

3 Stir in the garlic and all the spices and cook for a few minutes or until the aromas are released.

4 Add the tomatoes, apricots and stock, season with black pepper and stir to combine. Return the lamb to the casserole, bring to a gentle simmer and cover with a lid.

5 Transfer the casserole to the oven and cook for 1 hour. Check the lamb and, if it is still a little tough, cook for a further 20 minutes.

6 Serve with quinoa, sprinkled with coriander and toasted almonds.

*top tip

Slow-cooked stews and tagines are a great meal for mums as they cook in the oven while you take care of baby and last for several meals.

Grilled Cod Fillet with Papaya and Red Onion Relish

Serves 2

Ingredients

2 cod fillets

freshly ground black pepper

1 red onion, finely chopped

1 papaya, peeled and finely chopped

2 tablespoons chopped dill

juice and grated zest of 1 lime

1 courgette, sliced

Method

1 Preheat the grill to high.

2 Place the the fish on a baking tray, season with black pepper and grill for 8–10 minutes or until cooked, turning occasionally.

3 Meanwhile, mix the red onion, papaya and dill in a bowl and marinate in the lime juice and zest.

4 Arrange the courgette slices on 2 plates and place the fish on top. Spoon over the papaya and red onion relish and serve.

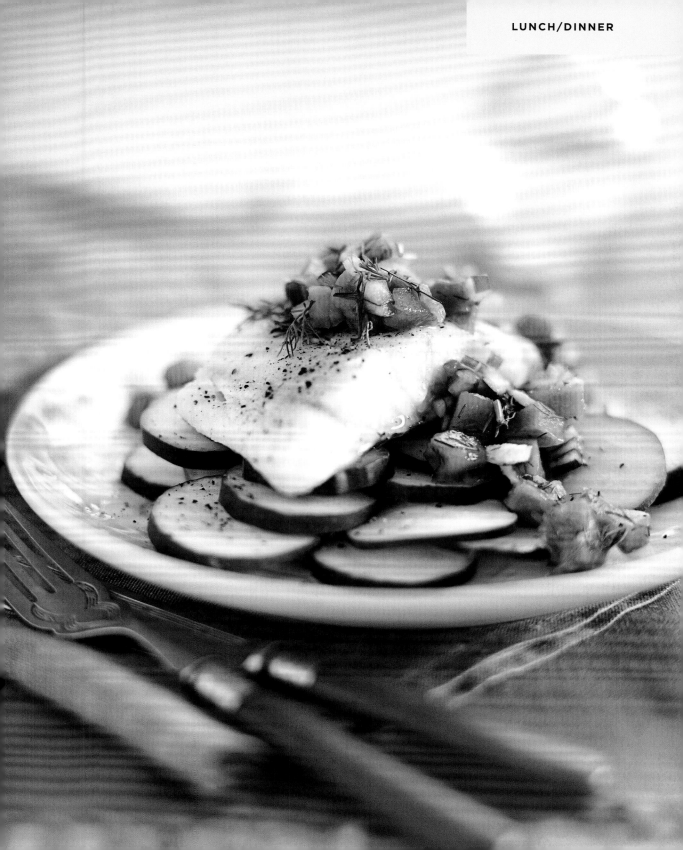

Hummus

Serves 4

Ingredients
250g dried chickpeas, soaked overnight in water
3–5 tablespoons lemon juice
1½ tablespoons tahini
2 garlic cloves, crushed
½ teaspoon sea salt
2 tablespoons extra virgin olive oil
toasted pitta bread, to serve

Method
1 Drain the soaked chickpeas, place in a saucepan, cover with fresh water, bring to the boil and simmer until soft. Drain, reserving the liquid, and allow to cool.

2 Combine the remaining ingredients, except the olive oil, in a food-processor. Add 120ml of the reserved chickpea liquid and blend until smooth.

3 Transfer to a serving bowl, make a well in the centre and pour over the olive oil.

4 Serve with toasted pitta bread.

*top tip

Beautiful, jewel-like pomegranate seeds brighten up any meal, plus they're high in vitamins and fibre and promote good heart health.

Chicken, Pomegranate and Feta salad

Serves 2

Ingredients
2 free-range chicken breasts
freshly ground black pepper
80g rocket
80g watercress
50g feta cheese, crumbled
seeds of 1 pomegranate
1 lime

Method
1 Preheat the grill to high.

2 Season the chicken breasts with black pepper, place on a roasting tray and grill for 10–15 minutes or until cooked, turning occasionally.

3 Meanwhile, divide the rocket and watercress between 2 bowls. Sprinkle with the crumbled feta and pomegranate seeds, then gently toss.

4 Slice the cooked chicken breasts thinly and add to the bowls. Squeeze the lime over the salad before serving.

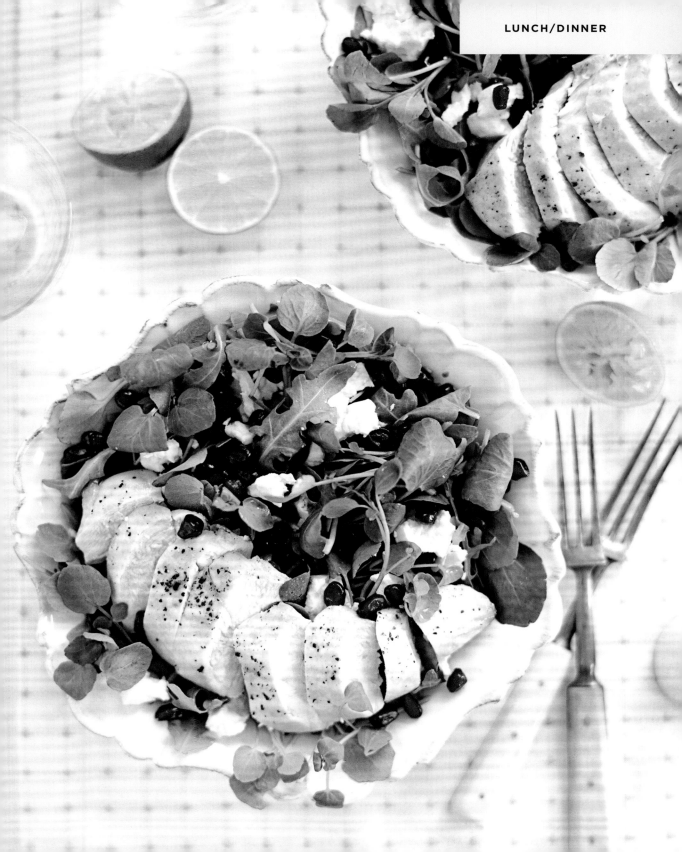

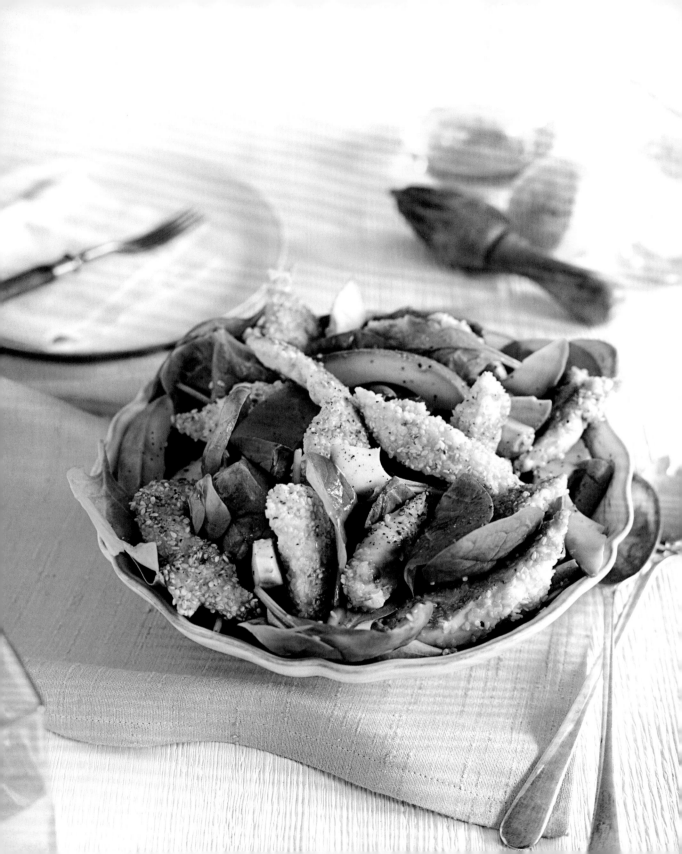

Sesame-crusted Chicken with Avocado and Spinach Salad

Serves 4

4 free-range chicken breasts, cut into 1cm strips
salt and freshly ground black pepper
3 tablespoons extra virgin olive oil
6 tablespoons sesame seeds
200g baby spinach leaves
1 avocado, peeled, stoned and sliced
For the dressing
2 tablespoons lemon juice
1 tablespoon extra virgin olive oil

Method

1 Season the chicken strips with salt and pepper.

2 Place 2 tablespoons of the olive oil in a bowl and scatter the sesame seeds over a large plate. Brush the chicken strips with olive oil and then roll in the sesame seeds to coat on both sides. Place the chicken on a sheet of baking parchment on a plate and refrigerate until needed.

3 Whisk the dressing ingredients together, season to taste and set aside.

4 Arrange the spinach leaves and avocado slices in a large bowl.

5 Heat a frying pan over a medium heat. When it is hot, add the remaining olive oil and then the sesame chicken strips. Fry the chicken until golden on one side before turning and cooking until golden on the other side.

6 As soon as the chicken is ready, add it to the spinach and avocado, drizzle over the dressing, toss to combine and serve.

*top tip

Avocados are full of fibre, vitamin K, folate, potassium and vitamin B6, as well as healthy monounsaturated fat. Teamed with nutrient-rich spinach and deliciously crunchy chicken for protein, they make a great salad.

Beef Stir-fry

Serves 2

Ingredients
80g spinach
80g mangetout
300g organic steak fillets, sliced into thin strips
freshly ground black pepper
1 garlic clove, finely chopped
1 teaspoon chopped fresh ginger
1 red chilli, finely chopped
60g spring onions, peeled and chopped
80g watercress
juice of 1 lime

Method

1 Place a wok on a high heat and stir-fry the spinach and mangetout for 3 minutes, or until softened.

2 Season the steak with black pepper and add to the pan, stir-frying until tender.

3 Add the garlic, ginger, chilli and spring onion to the wok and stir-fry for a further 2 minutes.

4 Serve the vegetables and beef on a bed of watercress, and drizzle with lime juice before serving.

*top tip

Oatcakes are one of the best snacks to have on hand when you're pregnant. They're tasty and filling and a great source of natural fibre.

Avocado and Salmon Oatcakes

Serves 2

Ingredients
1 ripe avocado, peeled, stoned and roughly chopped
4 plain organic oatcakes
100g smoked salmon
juice of 1 lemon
freshly ground black pepper

Method

1 Spread the avocado over the oatcakes.

2 Top with the smoked salmon, then drizzle with lemon juice and finish with a grind of black pepper.

Kale Crisps

Serves 4

Ingredients
200g kale
1 tablespoon olive oil
a pinch of sea salt

Method

1 Preheat the oven to 120°C/gas mark ½.

2 Remove the central stems from the kale and discard. Cut each leaf into pieces of about 10cm and toss them in a bowl with the olive oil and sea salt.

3 Spread the kale on a large baking tray in a single layer and bake in the oven for 30 minutes, or until crisp. Serve warm.

*top tip

Kale provides a useful dose of calcium plus vitamins A, C and K. And these are a great alternative to potato crisps – a common pregnancy craving – but without the saturated fat and much less salt.

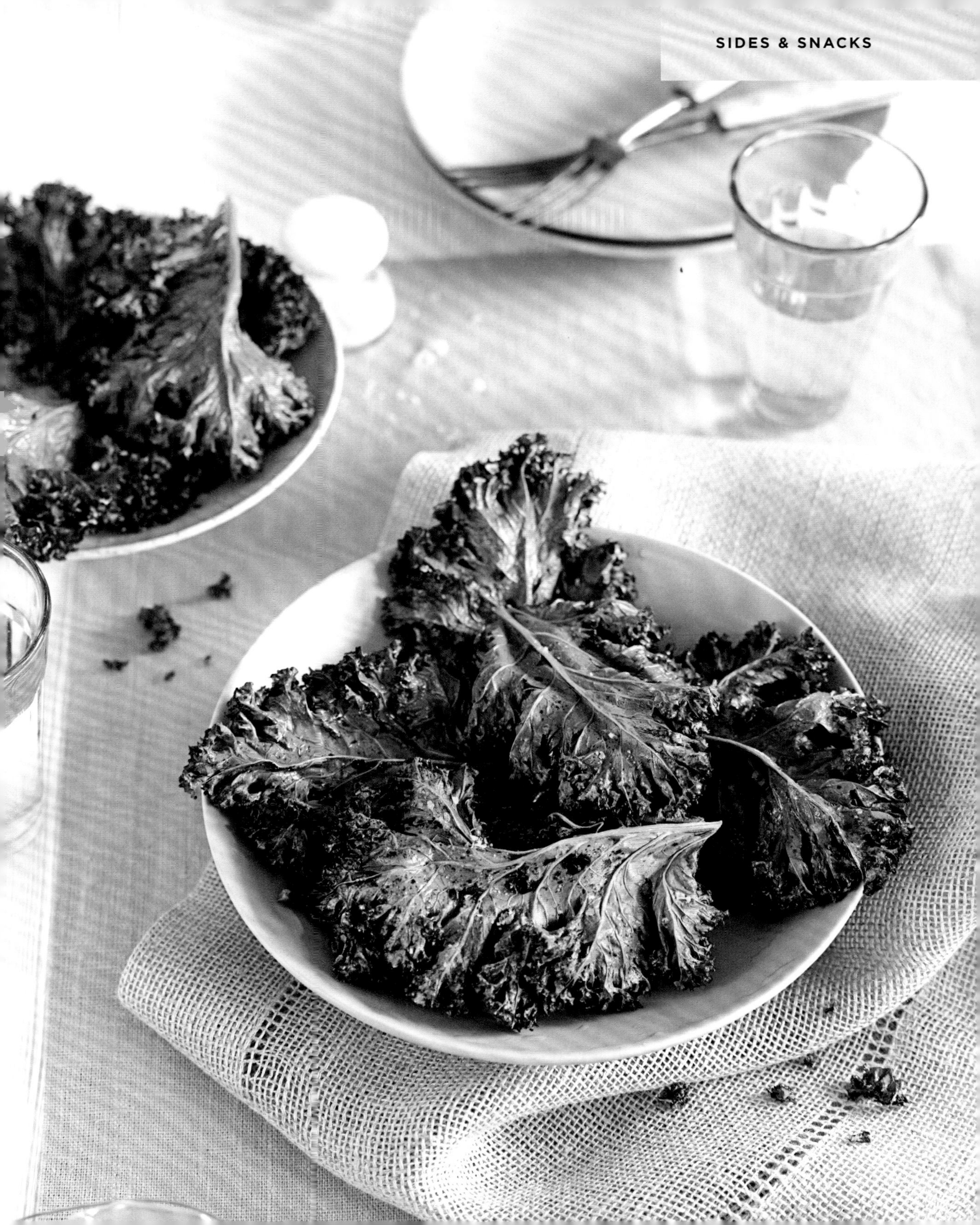

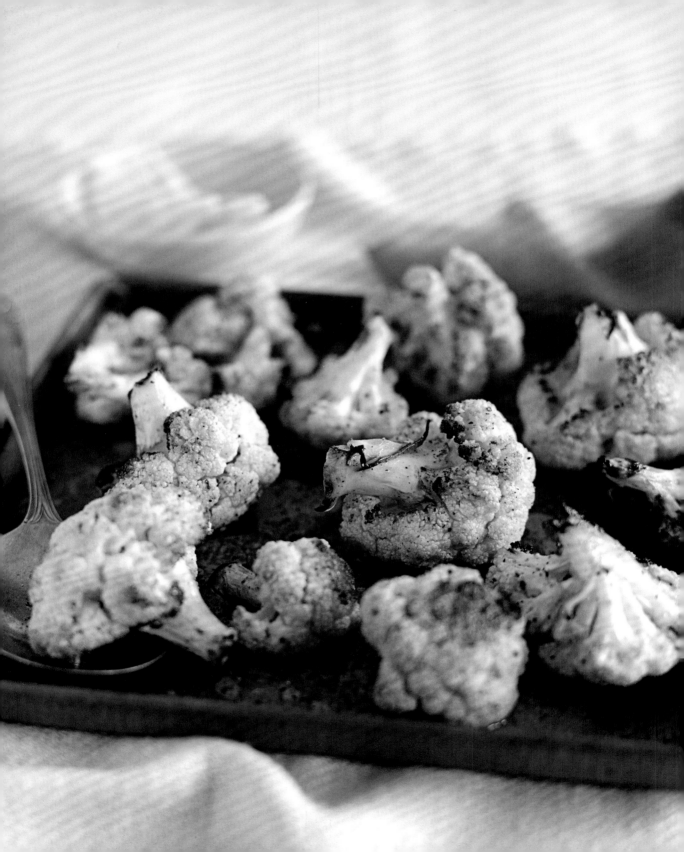

Roasted spiced cauliflower

Serves 4

Ingredients

1 head of cauliflower, broken into evenly sized florets
1 teaspoon ground cumin
1 tablespoon extra virgin olive oil
salt and freshly ground black pepper
squeeze of lemon juice, to serve (optional)

Method

1 Preheat the oven to 230°C/gas mark 8 and place the shelf in the lower third of the oven.

2 Place the cauliflower in a large bowl, add the cumin and drizzle over the olive oil. Toss well to coat the florets, and season with salt and pepper to taste.

3 Transfer the cauliflower to a baking tray and roast in the oven for about 25 minutes, turning once, until golden and tender.

4 Transfer to a serving bowl and serve, drizzled with a squeeze of lemon, if desired.

*top tip

This simple side dish is delicious and is a great accompaniment to fish or chicken – and cauliflower is an excellent source of dietary fibre, as well as vitamins C, K and B6.

Toasted Spelt Bread with Various Toppings

Add any of the following to some toasted spelt bread:

✳ Tuna, avocado, tomato, some freshly squeezed lime juice and a sprinkling of coriander leaves
✳ Poached eggs, steamed spinach and mushrooms
✳ Hummus, turkey and rocket

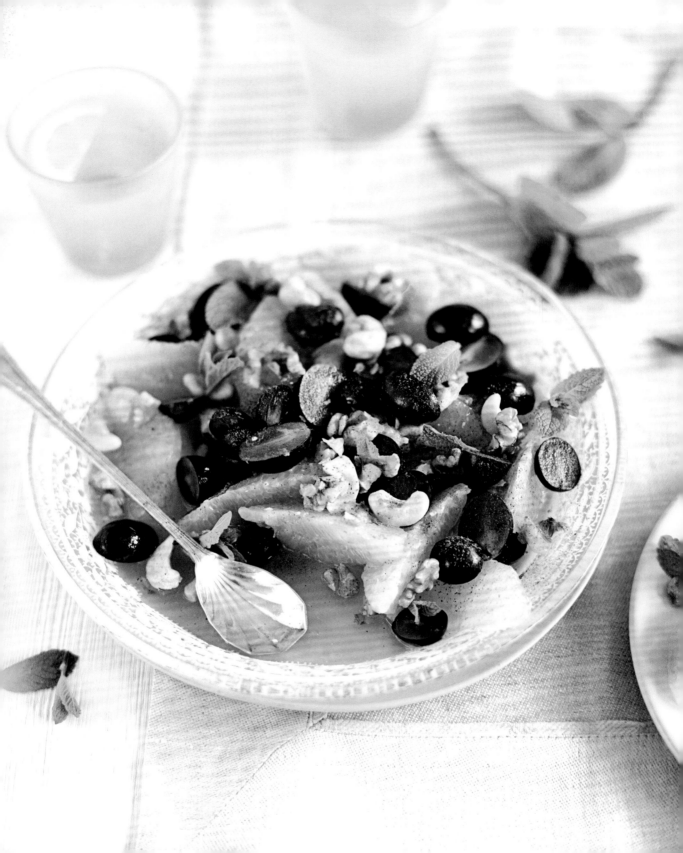

Pink Grapefruit and Black Grape Salad
Serves 2

Ingredients
2 pink grapefruit
125g black grapes, halved
1 tablespoon chopped walnuts
1 tablespoon cashew nuts
a handful of fresh mint leaves
1 teaspoon ground cinnamon

Method
1 Halve the grapefruit, remove all the peel and white pith, divide into segments and collect the juice in a bowl.

2 In 2 small serving bowls, mix the grapefruit segments and juice with the black grapes, walnuts and cashew nuts. Top with the mint leaves and ground cinnamon and serve.

*top tip
Christiane craved ice cream during her pregnancy because it was cold and sweet. So she blended mango, banana and avocado together and froze it – it makes life seem completely perfect, even if only for a few minutes!

Grilled Summer Peaches
Serves 2

Ingredients
4 peaches, halved and stoned
2 teaspoons manuka honey
6 tablespoons plain full-fat organic yogurt
150g blueberries
fresh mint leaves, roughly torn

Method
1 Preheat the grill to medium.

2 Place the peach halves on a baking tray and drizzle with the honey. Place the tray under the grill for 2–3 minutes, or until the peaches are warmed through.

3 Meanwhile, divide the yogurt between two serving dishes.

4 Place the warm peaches on top of the yogurt. Scatter the blueberries over the top and add the torn-up fresh mint leaves.

Apple and Blackberry Crumbles
Serves 2

Ingredients
50g rolled oats
50g almonds, chopped
2 tablespoons honey
3 apples, peeled, cored and cut into chunks
75ml organic apple juice
1 teaspoon ground cinnamon
150g blackberries

Method

1 Preheat the oven to 180°C/gas mark 4 and place the shelf in the middle.

2 Mix the oats, almonds and honey and spread over a baking tray. Place the tray in the oven and bake for 10–15 minutes, or until the mixture is golden brown.

3 Meanwhile, combine the apples, apple juice and cinnamon in a saucepan and allow to simmer for 10–15 minutes, or until the apples are soft. Stir in the blackberries.

4 Divide the apple and blackberry mixture between 2 serving dishes and sprinkle the oat and almond crumble mix over the top.

Lemon and Ginger Ice Lollies
Makes 8

Ingredients
475ml water
5cm piece of fresh ginger, peeled and chopped
25g caster sugar
125ml freshly squeezed lemon juice

Method

1 Put the water in a medium saucepan and place over a medium heat. Add the ginger and bring to a simmer, stirring occasionally. Remove from the heat, add the sugar, and stir until it has dissolved. Cover and leave to infuse for 10 minutes.

2 Add the lemon juice, stir and then strain into ice-lolly moulds. Freeze for 2–3 hours until completely frozen.

*top tip

These lollies are a great way to cool down if you're feeling overheated – a common complaint for pregnant women. Plus, as we know, the ginger eases nausea.

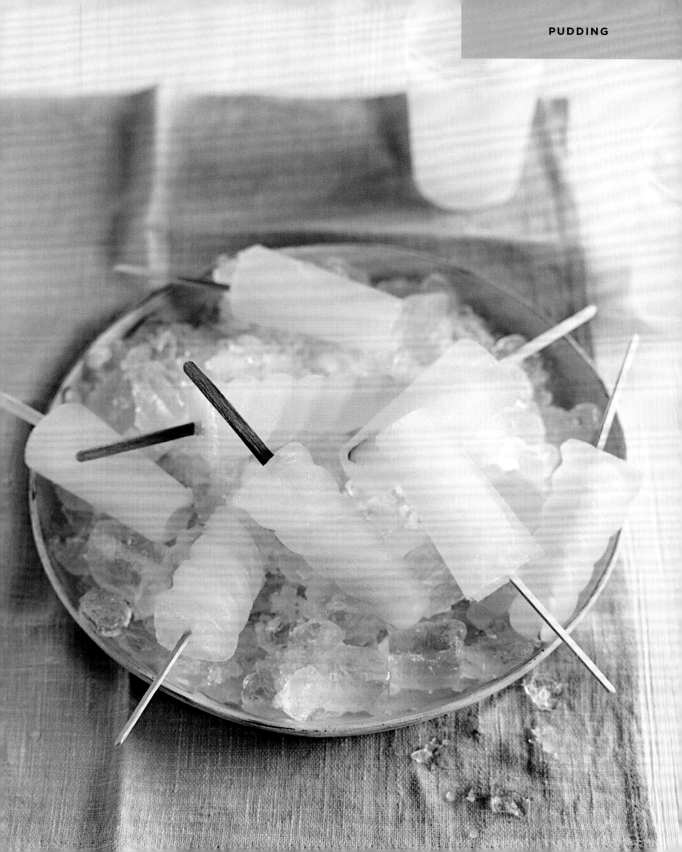

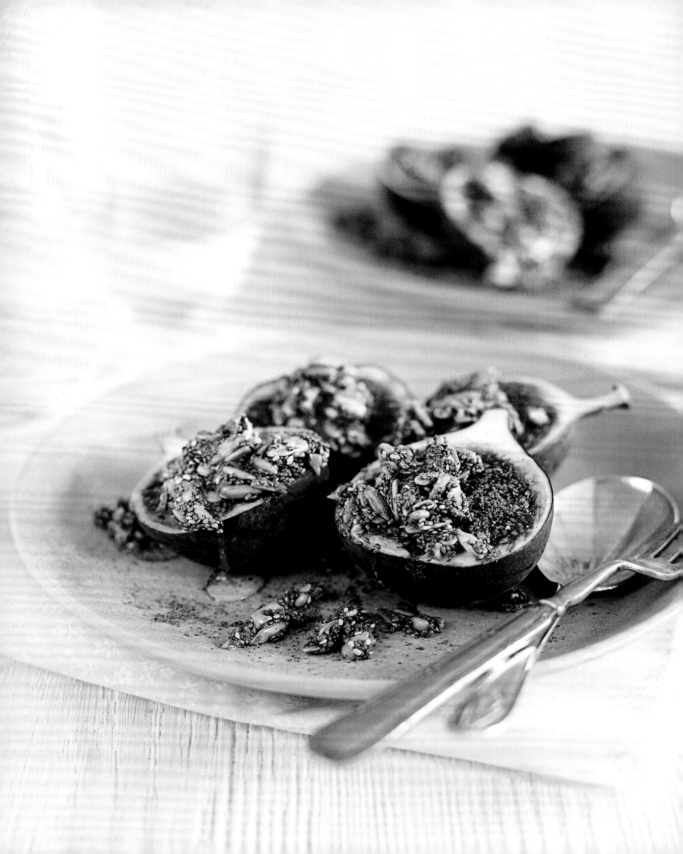

Figs with Chia Seeds

Serves 2

Ingredients
4 figs
50g chia seeds
50g sunflower seeds
2 tablespoons agave syrup
1 teaspoon grated nutmeg

Method
1 Halve the figs and arrange on 2 plates.

2 Mix the chia seeds and sunflower seeds together, using the agave syrup to bind them. Spread the seed mixture over the fig halves and dust with nutmeg.

*top tip
Chia seeds are a nutrient-dense source of protein and essential fatty acids. Scatter them over muesli, salads, stir-fries and puddings and whatever else takes your fancy.

Chocolate Fudge Tarts

Serves 4

Ingredients
For the tart cases
175g almonds
175g Medjool dates
1½ tablespoons melted coconut oil
1 tablespoon cocoa powder
a pinch of sea salt flakes
For the filling
2 large bananas, peeled
½ ripe avocado
30g cocoa powder
½ teaspoon ground cinnamon
1 tablespoon maple syrup
½ tablespoon water

Method
1 Blend all the ingredients for the tart cases in a food-processor until fine and crumbly. Taking 2 tablespoons of the mixture at a time, press into small muffin or tart cases, making sure there are no holes. Place in the freezer to set.

2 To make the filling, mix all the ingredients together in a blender for 30 seconds. Pour into the tart cases and place in the fridge to set for 30 minutes before serving.

PRE-PREGNANCY

If you're trying to get pregnant, try one of these fertility-boosting smoothies for breakfast or as a snack.

Refreshing Smoothie

Ingredients

240ml coconut water (and coconut flesh, if available; don't worry if you can't get the flesh though – bottled coconut water from a supermarket or health-food store is fine)

½ peach, peeled and stoned

1 scoop Clean & Lean Beauty Food*

a small handful of cashew nuts

¼ teaspoon ground cinnamon

3 ice cubes

1 teaspoon flaxseed oil

Method

Blend all the ingredients together and serve immediately.

Brilliant Smoothie

Ingredients

200ml rice or almond milk or coconut water

1 scoop Clean & Lean Body Brilliance*

½ teaspoon ground cinnamon

5 Brazil nuts

4 fresh mint leaves

2 ice cubes

Method

Blend all the ingredients together and serve immediately.

Essential Smoothie

Ingredients

200ml rice or almond milk or coconut water

1 scoop Clean & Lean Body Brilliance*

1 scoop Clean & Lean Beauty Food*

½ banana

1 tablespoon coconut oil

1 teaspoon chia seeds

Method

Blend all the ingredients together and serve immediately.

Baby-making Shake for Men

Ingredients

a large handful of your favourite leafy greens

1 carrot, peeled

200ml pomegranate juice

a small handful of Brazil nuts

a small handful of pumpkin seeds

1cm fresh ginger

a large handful of ice

Method

Blend all the ingredients together and serve immediately.

Male Testo Shake

Ingredients

200ml rice or almond milk or coconut water

1 scoop Clean & Lean Male Testo*

4 Brazil nuts

a small handful of pumpkin seeds

a small handful of berries of your choice

Method

Blend all the ingredients together and serve immediately.

BUMP-FRIENDLY

If you're pregnant, try one of these smoothies packed with Clean & Lean goodness for you and your baby.

Nourishing Smoothie

Ingredients

½ avocado, peeled and stoned

½ banana

a large handful of blueberries

1 teaspoon chia seeds

ice

Method

Blend all the ingredients together and serve immediately.

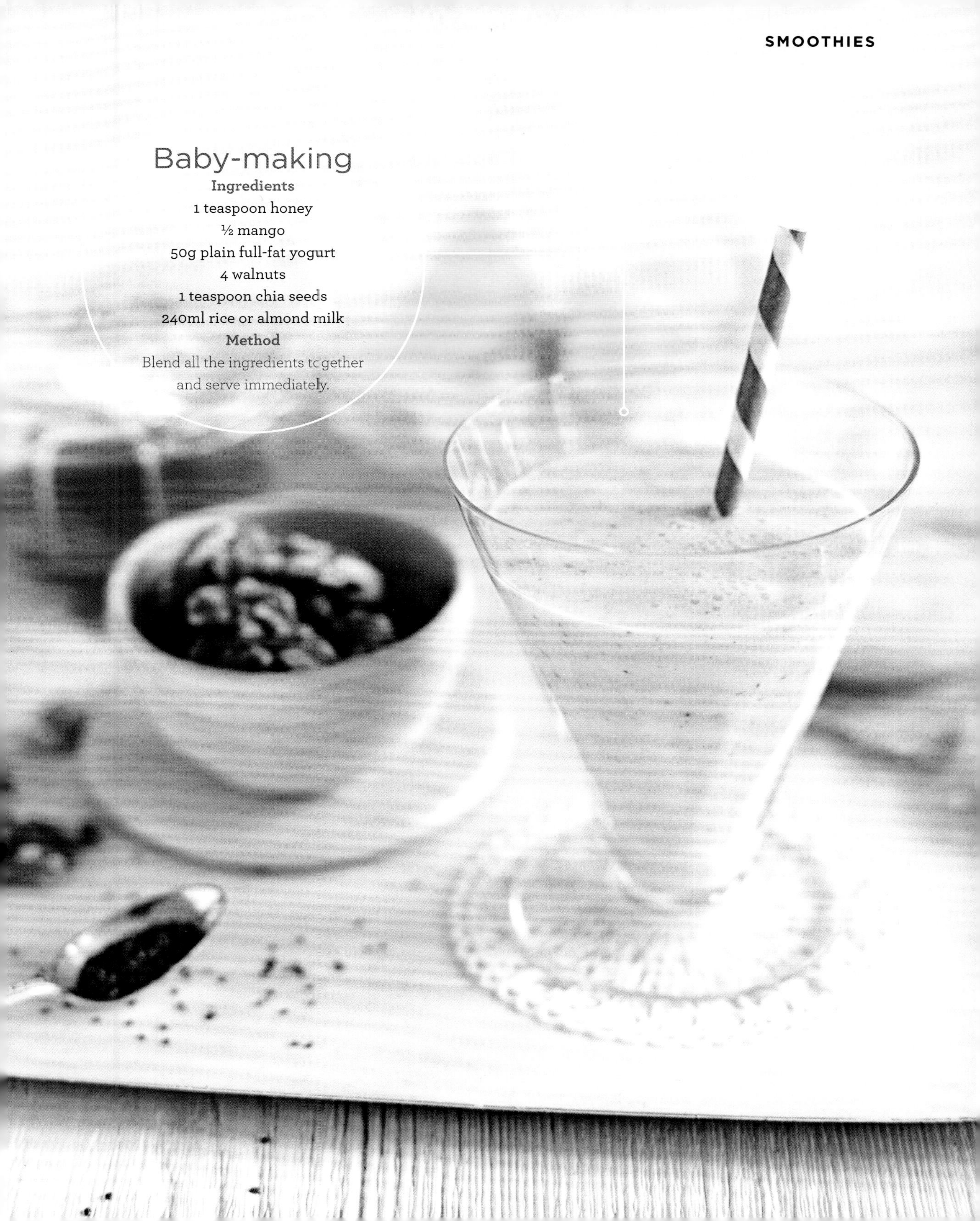

Baby-making

Ingredients

1 teaspoon honey

½ mango

50g plain full-fat yogurt

4 walnuts

1 teaspoon chia seeds

240ml rice or almond milk

Method

Blend all the ingredients together
and serve immediately.

Crave-quench Juice

Ingredients
a small handful of raspberries
3 fresh mint leaves
juice of ½ lime
sparkling water
ice

Method
Blend all the ingredients together and serve immediately.

Refreshing Juice

Ingredients
½ watermelon, peeled
3 fresh mint leaves
a small piece of fresh ginger
ice

Method
Blend all the ingredients together and serve immediately.

Hydrating Smoothie

Ingredients
a handful of broccoli florets
1 celery stick
1 pear, peeled and cored
juice of ½ lemon
a few fresh mint leaves
ice

Method
Blend all the ingredients together and serve immediately.

Pick-me-up

Ingredients
1 carrot, peeled
1 celery stick
1 apple, peeled and cored
a small piece of fresh ginger, peeled
juice of 1 lime
ice

Method
Blend all the ingredients together and serve immediately.

Ruby Green Smoothie

Ingredients

1 green apple, cored

a small piece of fresh ginger

1 teaspoon ground cinnamon

a large handful of spinach leaves

a large handful of kale leaves

1 teaspoon bee pollen

1 tablespoon chia seeds

ice (or add water as you like, for thickness)

Method

Blend all the ingredients together and serve immediately.

Vitamin Kick

Ingredients

a small handful of beetroot, peeled and chopped

$1/3$ cucumber

1 green pepper, deseeded

a large handful of raspberries

Method

Blend all the ingredients together and serve immediately.

Calming Evening Shake

Ingredients

240ml almond milk

a small handful of cashew nuts

½ banana

a pinch of ground cinnamon

Method

Blend all the ingredients together and serve immediately.

Coconut and Berry Smoothie

Ingredients

150g Coyo (coconut yogurt)

1 banana

a pinch of coconut flakes

a handful of raspberries

1 teaspoon honey

Method

Blend all the ingredients together and serve immediately.

POST-BABY

If you're a new mum increase your energy levels with one of these Clean & Lean new-mum smoothies.

Bedtime Smoothie

Ingredients

200ml rice milk, milk or water

1 scoop Clean & Lean Serenity*

½ teaspoon ground cinnamon

2 ice cubes

4 fresh mint leaves

Method

Blend all the ingredients together and serve immediately

Rejuvenating Smoothie

Ingredients

200ml coconut water

1 scoop Clean & Lean Beauty Food*

2 ice cubes

4 fresh mint leaves

a small handful of spinach

a handful of blueberries

Method

Blend all the ingredients together and serve immediately

Fat-burning Smoothie

Ingredients

200ml coconut water

1 scoop Clean & Lean Berry Burn*

5–6 raspberries

4 fresh mint leaves

2 ice cubes

Method

Blend all the ingredients together and serve immediately.

*top tip

*All Clean & Lean products are available at bodyism.com

{ Afterword }

by Christy Turlington

founder of Every Mother Counts

Taking good care of your health before and during pregnancy is the most important thing a mother can do for her child. Eating a clean diet and getting enough exercise and rest was a big part of why I felt so strong and powerful going into my first pregnancy. I knew what kind of birth I wanted, so I found a doula (somebody who supports the mother in her pregnancy, birth and early parenthood in a practical and emotional, but non-medical way) who helped to prepare me and put a team in place. My husband supported me all the way through and participated as much as any partner could. Together we decided which midwife to work with and that helped determine where we would deliver.

It was the middle of winter when we learned that we would be parents, so it was a perfect time to nest and start planning. The changes my body went through were wonderful and I celebrated them all. I pored over books about pregnancy and parenting and happily slowed my work schedule down a notch or two because I could. I continued to practise yoga right up to the day before I went into labour.

It was late October when I went into labour with my first baby, my daughter Grace. My doula

> *Every Mother Counts is a campaign to end preventable deaths caused by pregnancy and childbirth around the world.*

and my husband helped me get through the early hours at home. By the time I went to the birth centre to meet up with my midwife, I was in hard labour. With the help of my 'dream team,' as I called them, I got my wish to have a natural birth. Grace was born exactly the way I'd hoped she would be and I was beyond happy to have her in my arms at long last. Then everything changed in a heartbeat.

There were complications with my placenta and I haemorrhaged. I went from feeling powerful to being powerless, from being exhilarated to being scared. My midwife called in an obstetrician, who was in my room in a matter of seconds. The midwife and doctor worked together seamlessly to stop the bleeding and save my life. What would have happened if they had not been there?

That question stayed on my mind during my early months as a mother. I've travelled all over the world throughout my career as a model and I've seen the spectrum of care that pregnant women receive, or don't in many cases. Often, there is no medical care, let alone running water or skilled midwives and doctors, no transportation to get to the closest hospital and no power or money to facilitate women's own access to lifesaving medical care. I knew what the answer to my question would be: if I had given birth in any number of places around the world, I would have died. That's what motivated me to learn more about what happens when a woman does not have access to critical care. I learned that, at that time, half a million mothers died every year, many from the same complication as I had.

I decided to use my resources to document the conditions that cause these deaths and spent the next two years filming in Guatemala, Bangladesh, Tanzania and the United States. In 2010 I debuted my first documentary film, *No Woman, No Cry*, which examines some of the barriers that put millions of mothers at risk each year. My hope was that mothers could connect with other mothers through these universal stories about birth and be moved to join me so that together we could make pregnancy and childbirth safe for all mums. And that was the impetus of Every Mother Counts.

Every Mother Counts is a campaign to end preventable deaths caused by pregnancy and childbirth around the world. We inform, engage and mobilise new audiences to take action to improve the health and wellbeing of girls and women worldwide.

> *We need more people demanding that motherhood be respected so that more women can enjoy safe, supported pregnancies and deliveries.*

In the years since *No Woman, No Cry* was completed there has been a significant reduction in deaths in childbirth globally. With the effort of many individuals and organisations the estimates have been halved. We don't need new cures or treatments because we know how to save most of these lives. We need more families to know that this remains a problem in the 21st century. We need more people demanding that motherhood be respected so that more women can enjoy safe, supported pregnancies and deliveries and so these daunting statistics will continue declining at a steady rate.

Thank you, James and Christiane, for your commitment to mothers and the people who love them. By sharing the important information in this book, more women will achieve optimum health before, during and after pregnancy. By donating a portion of each e-book sold to Every Mother Counts, they also help ensure that more mothers around the world will have access to the critical care they may need when they give birth.

To learn more about Every Mother Counts and its mission to improve maternal health, visit www.everymothercounts.org

{INDEX}

{ Acknowledgements }

It's more than thank you. I don't even think there is a word to describe how grateful I feel to so many people. To Chrissy – it's all you. My heart is full up with you and our beautiful children. You are my best and most wonderful and I love you more than forever. To my brothers, Lee Mullins – finally you are an international model/celebrity. I love you so much. The sky is the limit for you, my brother. I've watched you grow into a spectacular man and I'm so proud of you. To David de Rothschild, for believing in me and standing with me through everything. To Teresa Palmer and Mark Webber for being so beautiful and for being love wherever we see you. To Luke and Chantal and Sienna and Jake and Sol... We love you so much. You bring strength, beauty, love and kindness into our lives and you are the best friends anyone could ever hope for. To my mama – thank you for being my mama and for raising me to be respectful and kind. To my papa, Kevin Duigan... You are the best of everything. You taught me to be kind and generous and strong. Anything good I've ever done is because of you. To my sister Ruby – I'm so proud of you. Thank you for being my best friend. To Angela Duigan for being more incredible than words can ever say and to all of our family for teaching us what it means to be truly loved and supported. To my cousin Ben, jorts or not, you are the strongest and kindest. Thank you Peter, Helo, Biela and Glenn – you are so generous with your love, time and energy for us and for Charlotte. Thank you surrounding us in pure love and joy. To Justin Alexander. Words won't suffice so let's just say... You're stronger and more amazing than anyone will ever know.. But I know. To the following angels in our lives – Lara Stone, Christy Turlington, Megan Gale – for beautiful words and beautiful bikinis. Holly Candy – is there anyone more loyal and wonderful than you? Sally Obermeder, so full of love and light. To those who were with us to guide and support every step of our journey: Emma Cannon, Ana Cannon, Claire Hamilton, Gemma Ireland. To Jay McGavigan, Julie Schiller, Jane Lyttleton – you brought the biggest treasure into our lives in the most loving, peaceful way possible and now are helping others to do the same through this book – THANK YOU. To Hani, for believing when nobody else could see, for being the bravest and kindest. To my second family at Bodyism: Hamish, Adena, Nat, Mike, Tegan, Jamie, Tom, Dmitri, Rebecca, Toby, Chris, Albert, Una, Wenche, Danai - you're the best (looking) team in the world and the reason why anything ever happens.

And finally to God, for all the miracles.

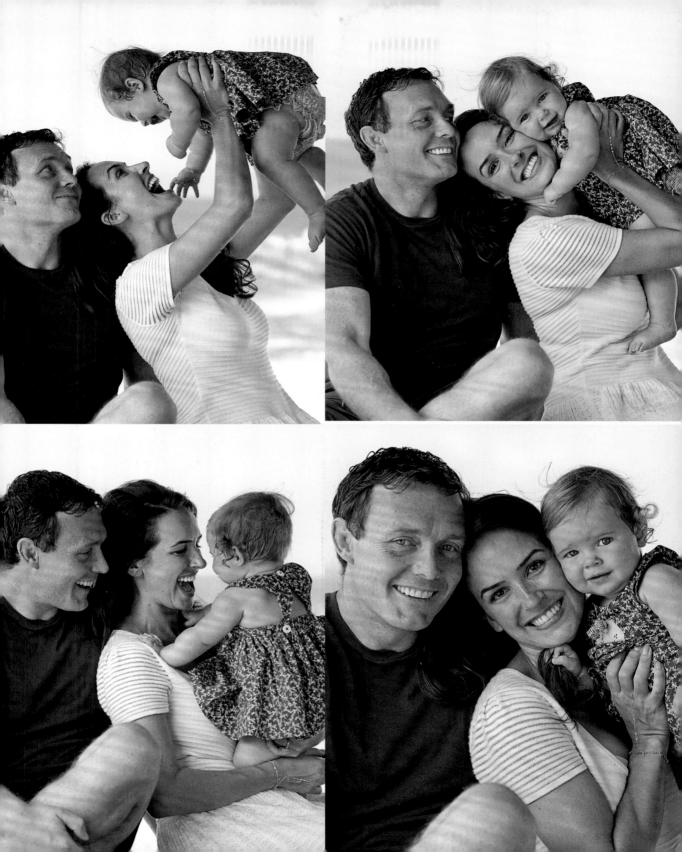

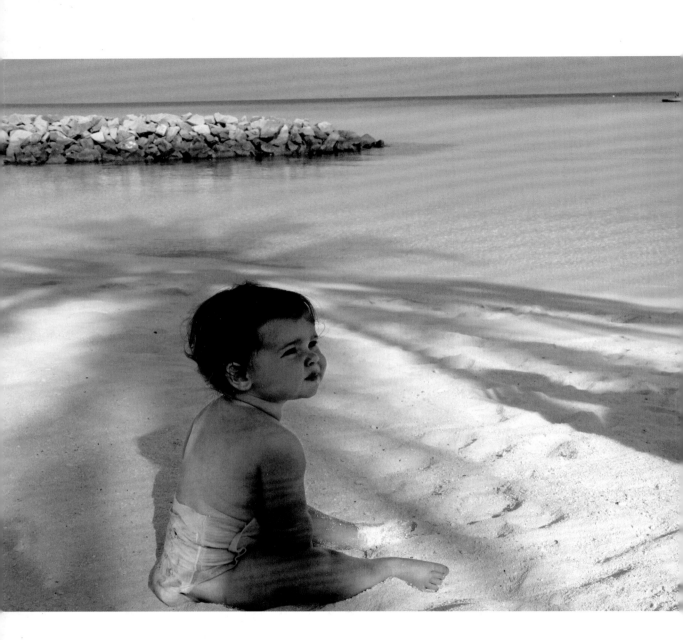

Here is a nice mantra to help in moments of doubt. Repeat after me 'love and gratitude'. Say it in time with your breathing. You'll feel better after even a minute.

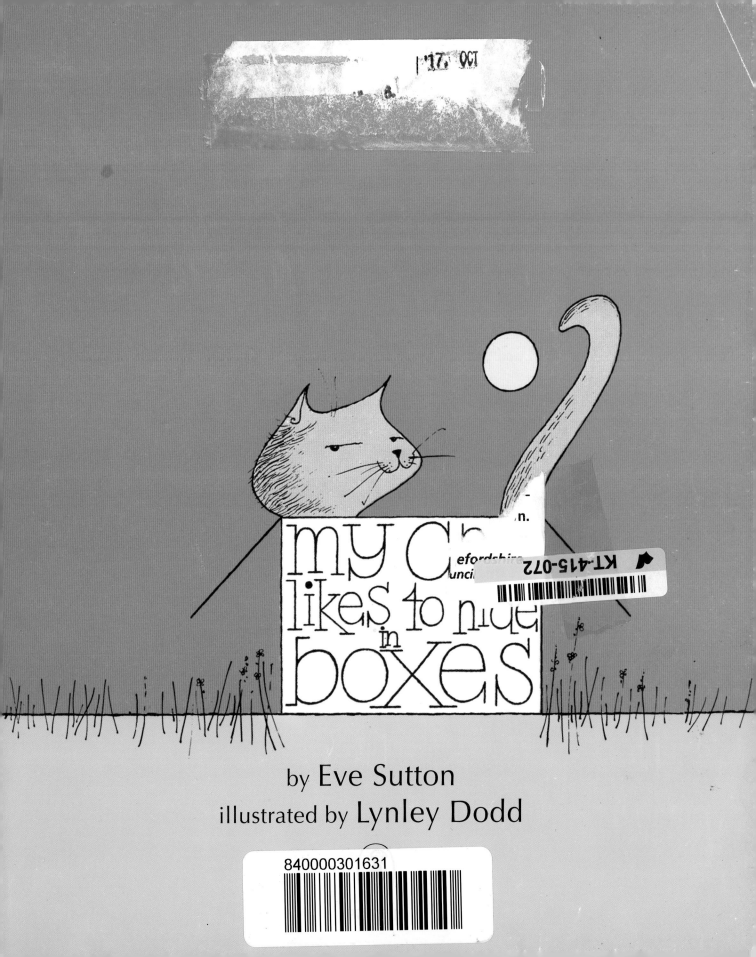

my cat likes to hide in boxes

by Eve Sutton
illustrated by Lynley Dodd

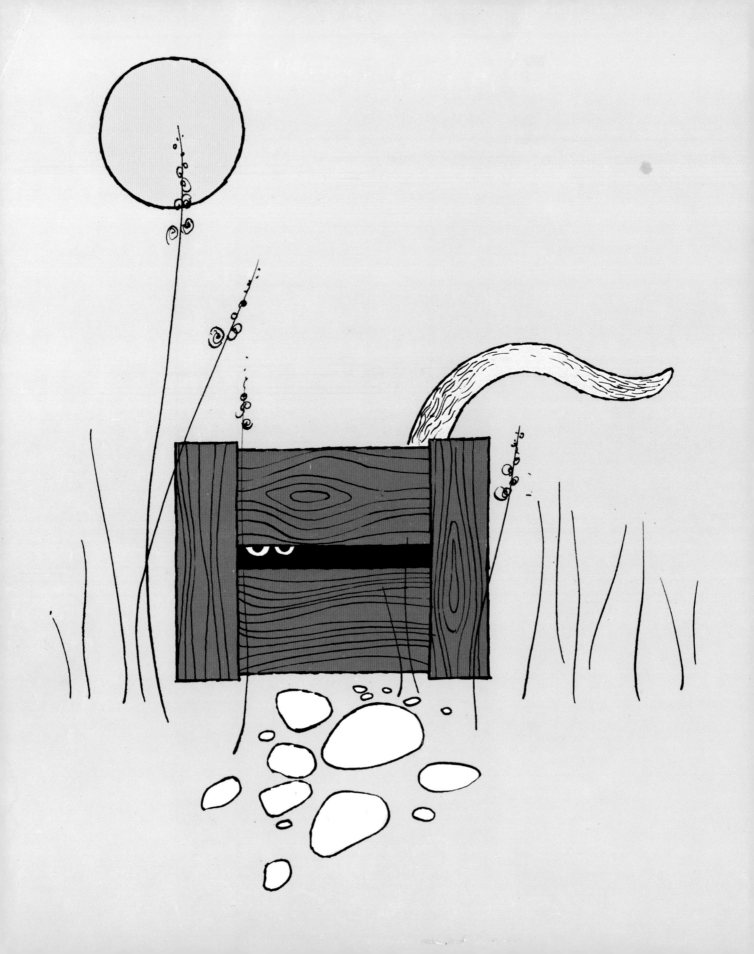

My cat likes to hide in boxes.

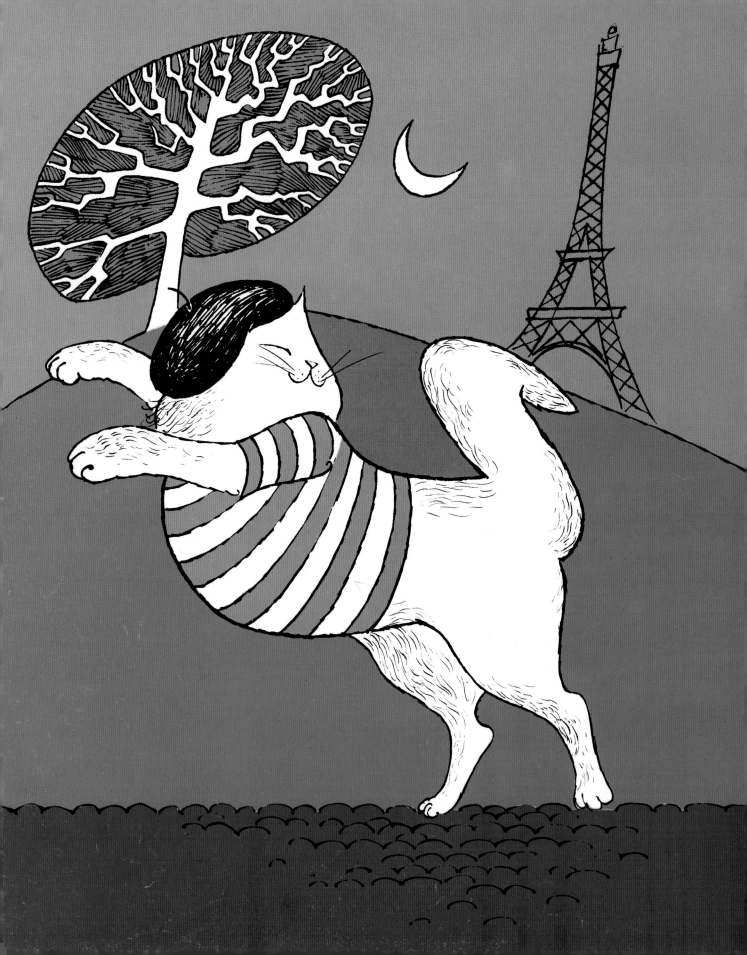

The cat from France
liked to sing and dance.

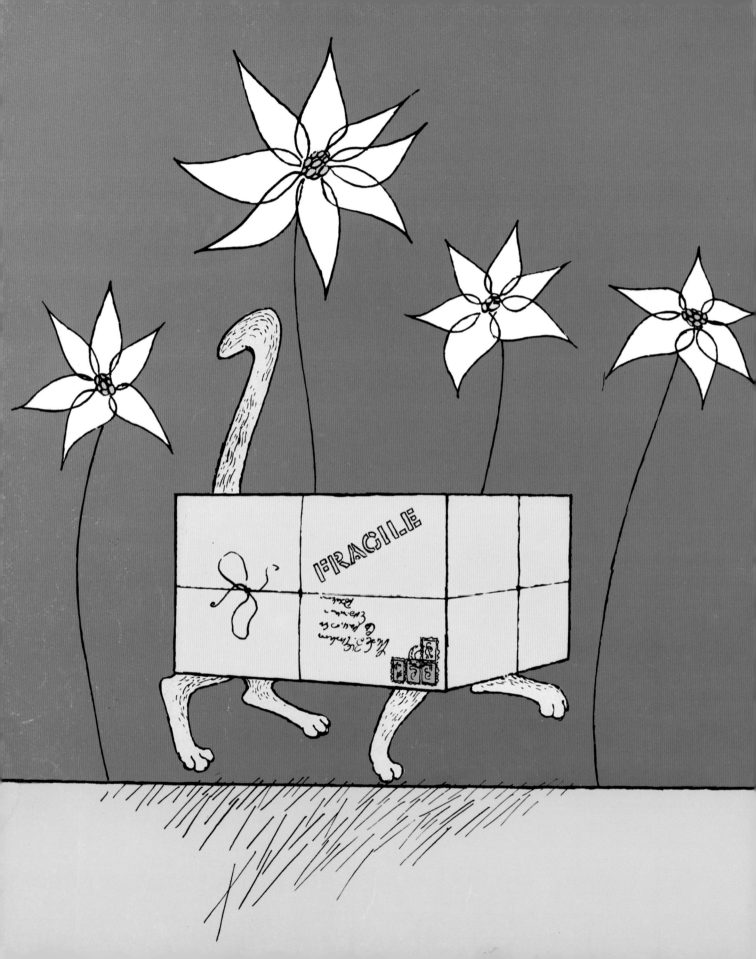

But MY cat likes to hide in boxes.

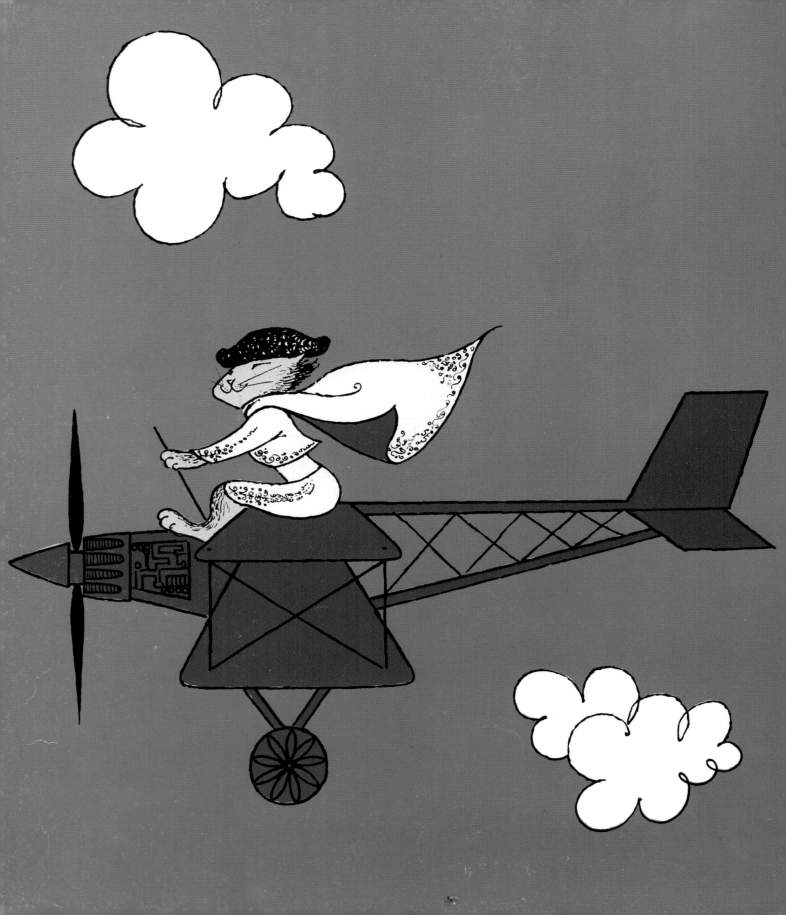

The cat from Spain
flew an aeroplane.
The cat from France
liked to sing and dance.

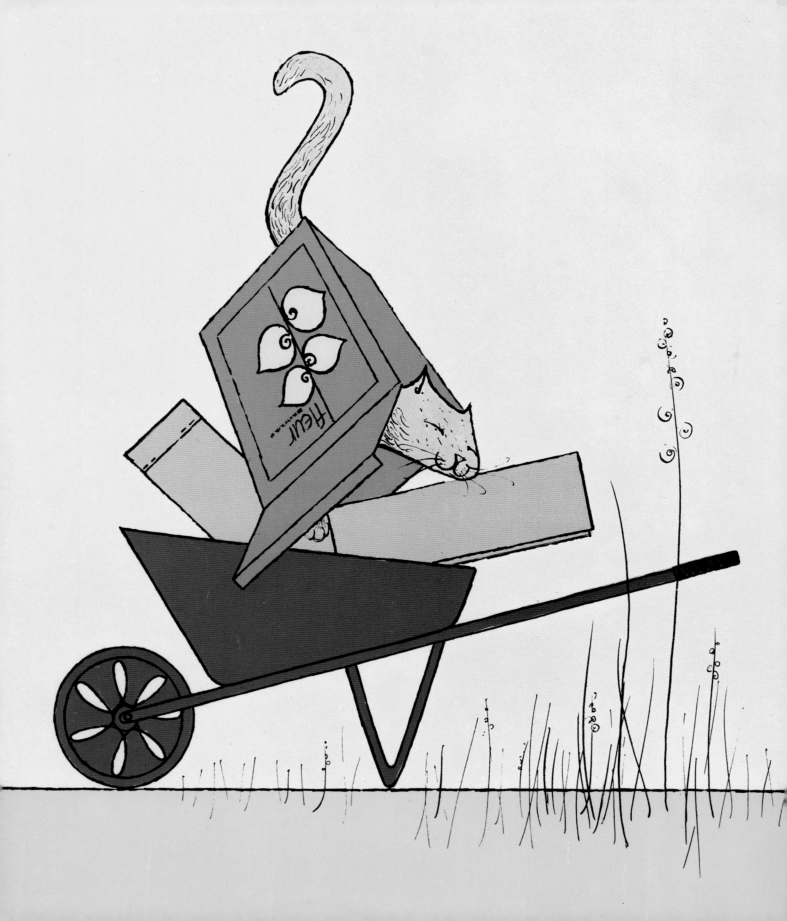

But MY cat likes to hide in boxes.

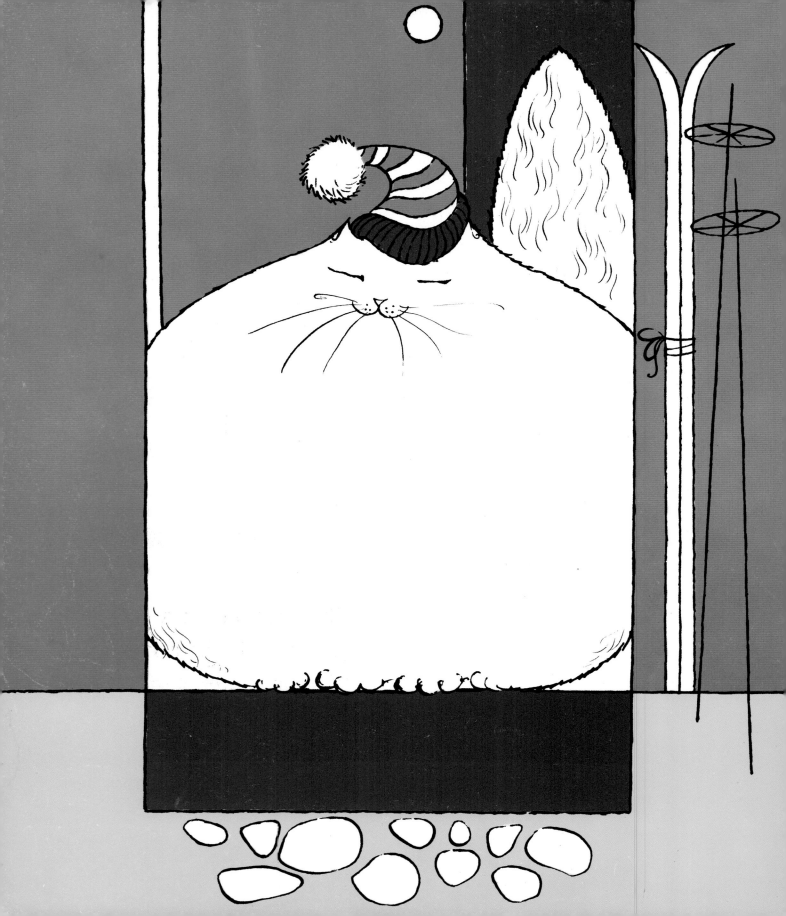

The cat from Norway
got stuck in the doorway.
The cat from Spain
flew an aeroplane.
The cat from France
liked to sing and dance.

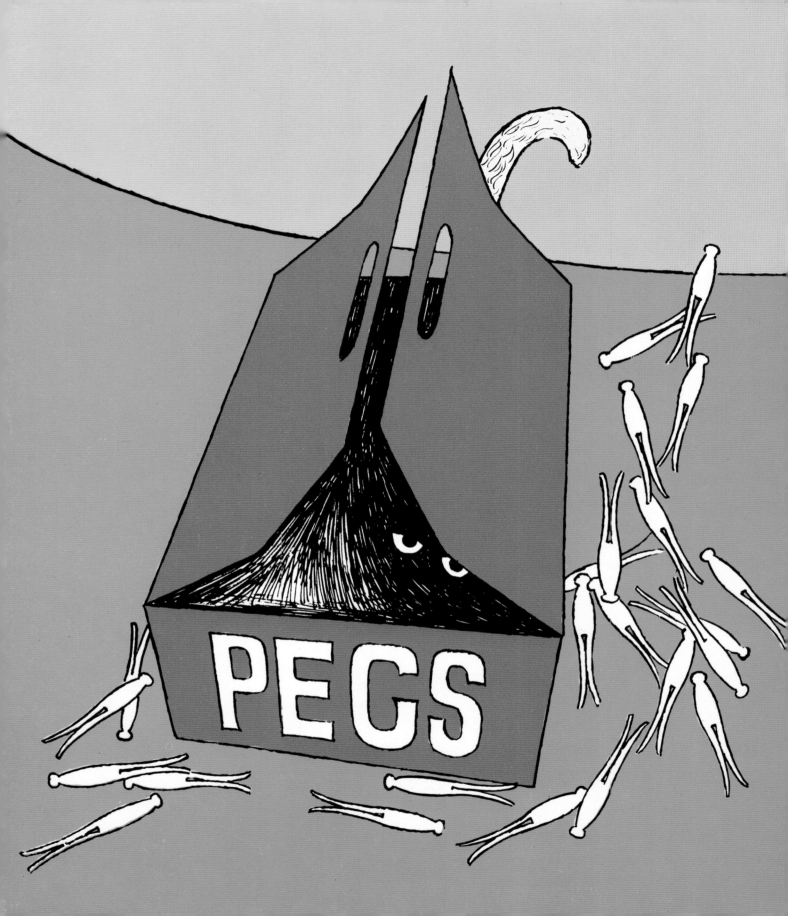

But MY cat likes to hide in boxes.

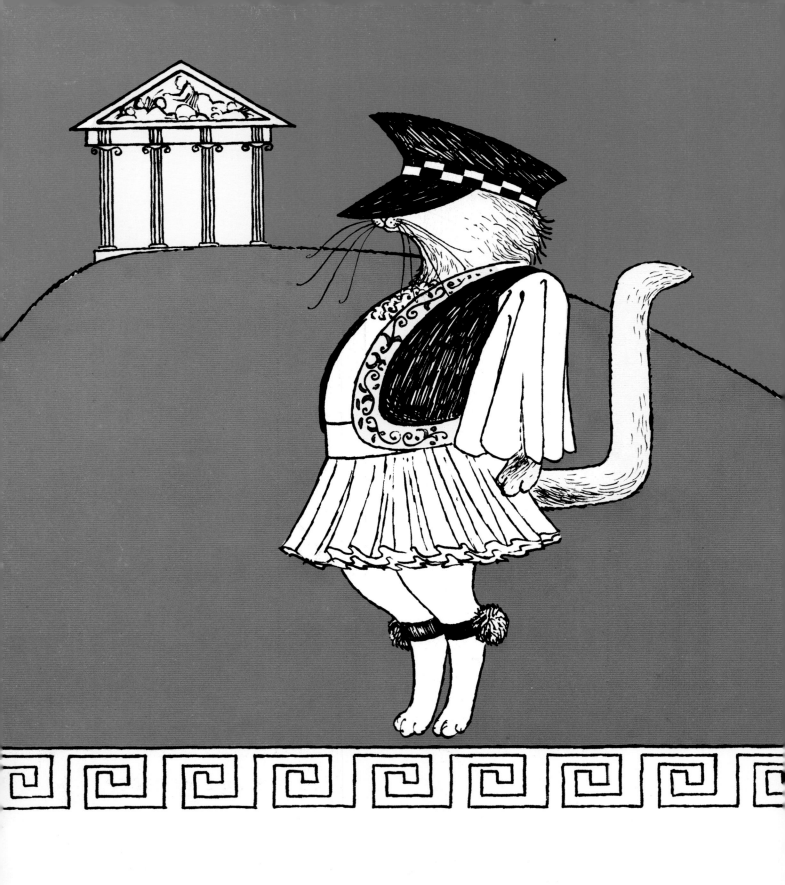

The cat from Greece
joined the police.
The cat from Norway
got stuck in the doorway.
The cat from Spain
flew an aeroplane.
The cat from France
liked to sing and dance.

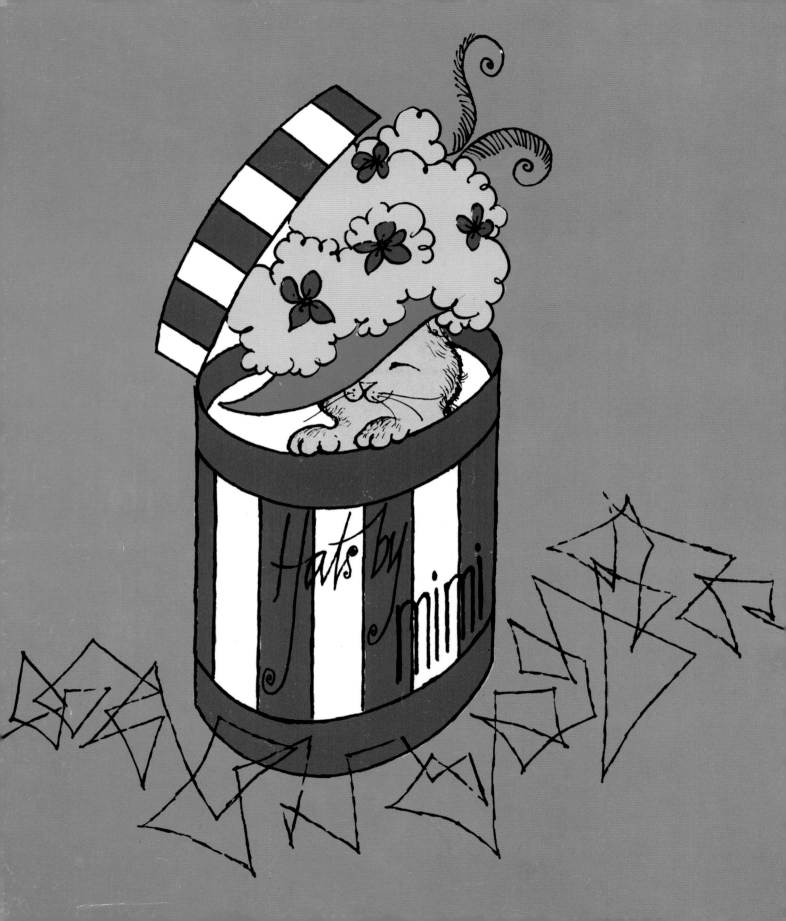

But MY cat likes to hide in boxes.

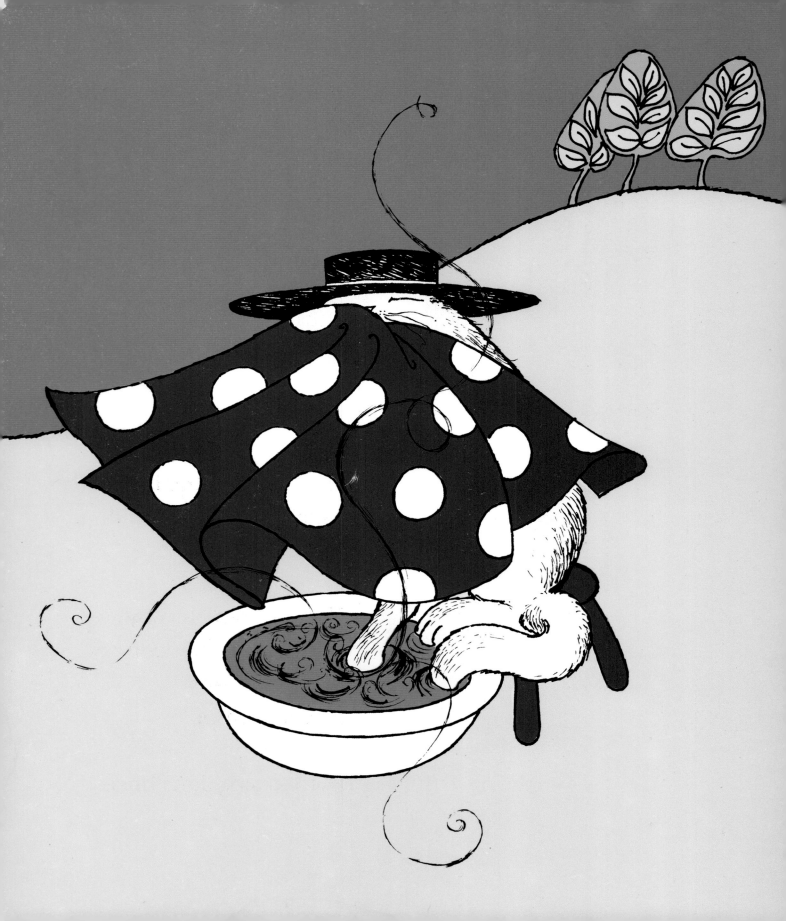

The cat from Brazil
caught a very bad chill.
The cat from Greece
joined the police.
The cat from Norway
got stuck in the doorway.
The cat from Spain
flew an aeroplane.
The cat from France
liked to sing and dance.

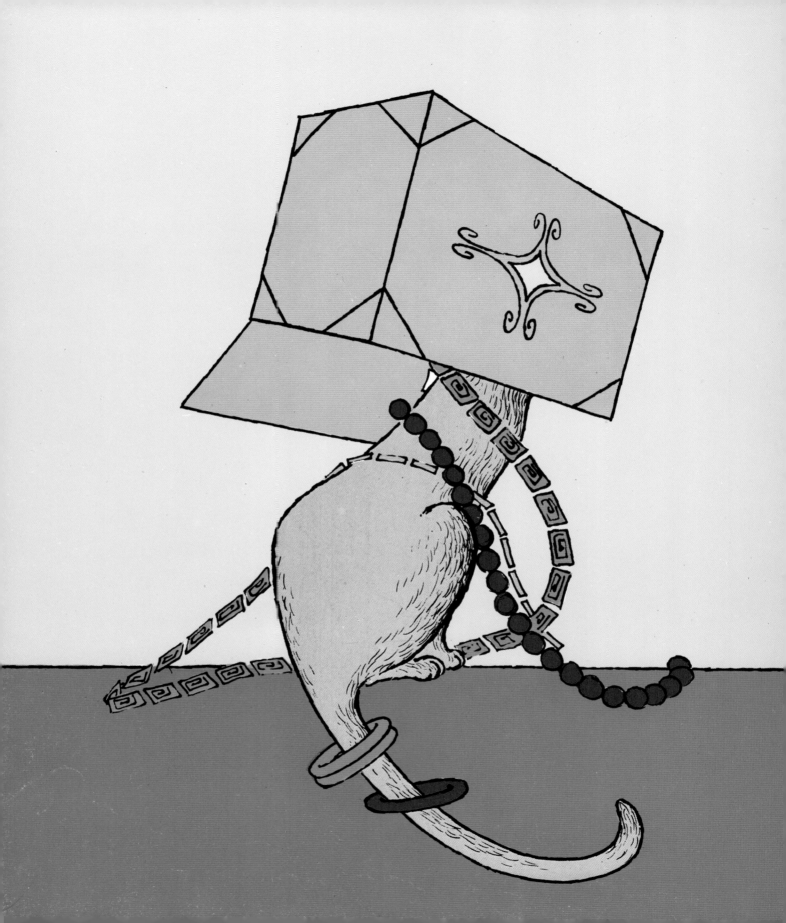

But MY cat likes to hide in boxes.

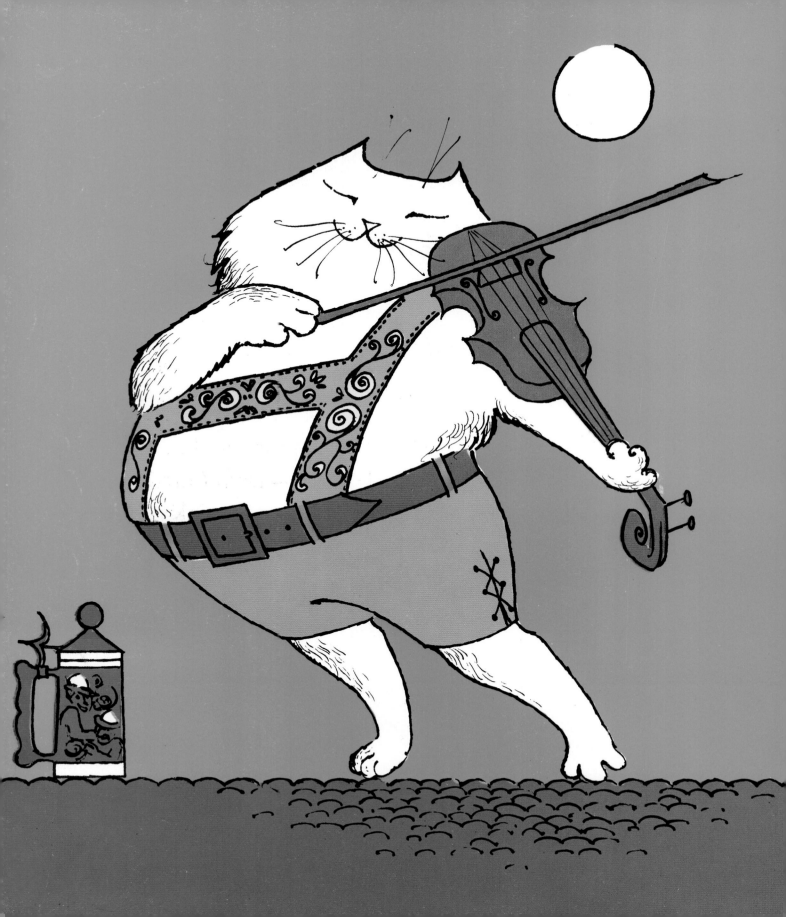

The cat from Berlin
played the violin.
The cat from Brazil
caught a very bad chill.
The cat from Greece
joined the police.
The cat from Norway
got stuck in the doorway.
The cat from Spain
flew an aeroplane.
The cat from France
liked to sing and dance.

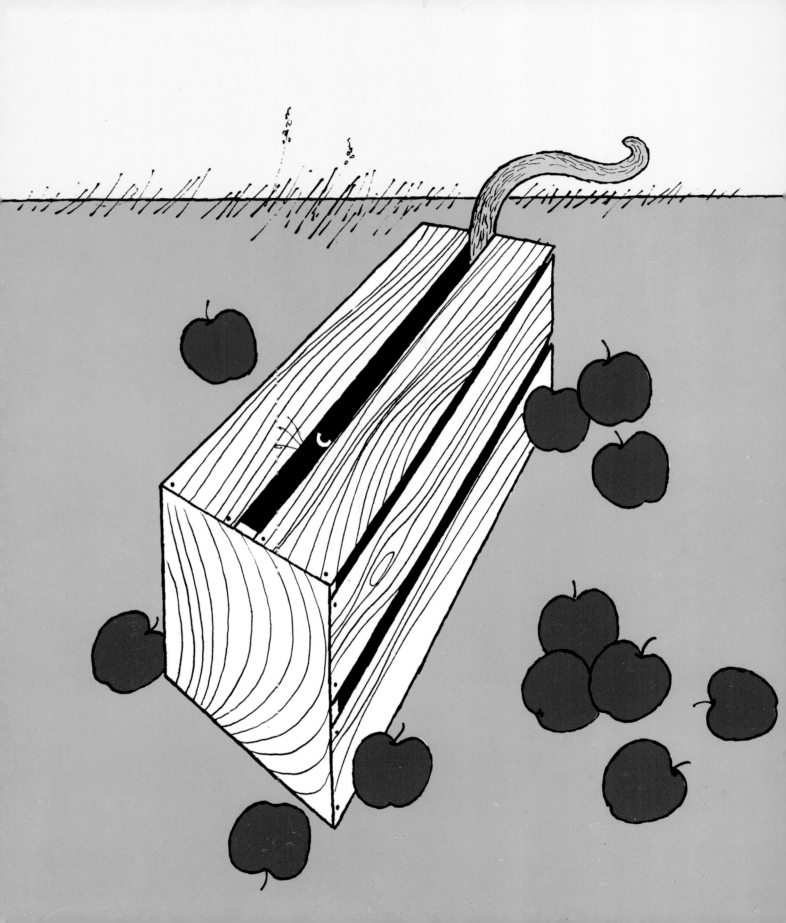

But MY cat likes to hide in boxes.

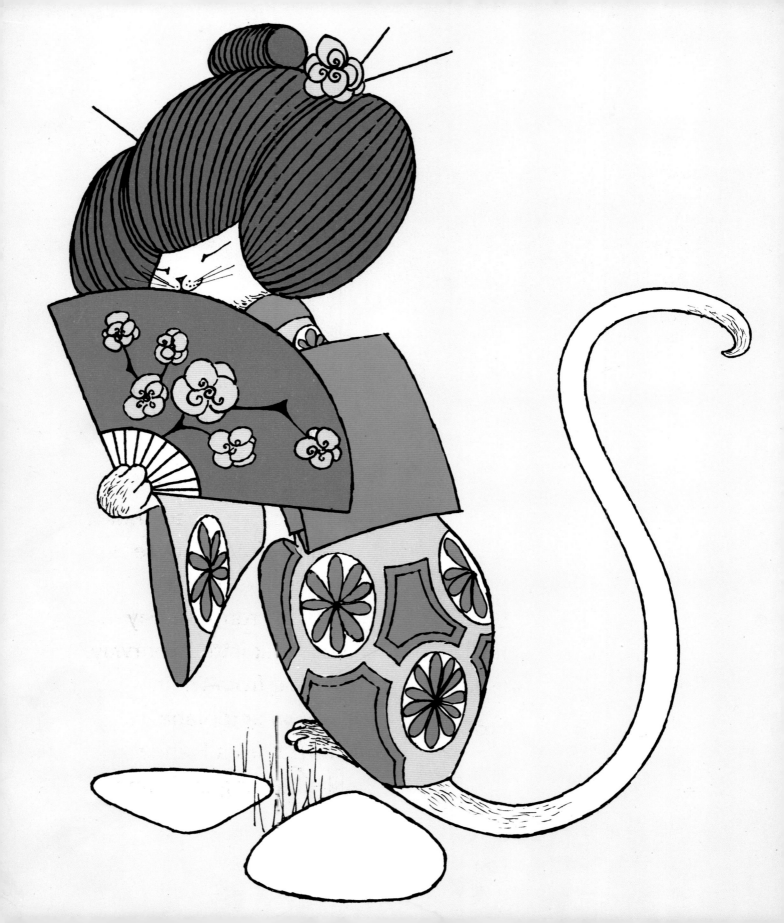

The cat from Japan
waved a big blue fan.
The cat from Berlin
played the violin.
The cat from Brazil
caught a very bad chill.
The cat from Greece
joined the police.
The cat from Norway
got stuck in the doorway.
The cat from Spain
flew an aeroplane.
The cat from France
liked to sing and dance.

Look at all these clever cats,
cats from Spain, Brazil and France,
cats from Greece, Japan and Norway,
cats who sing and fly and dance . . .

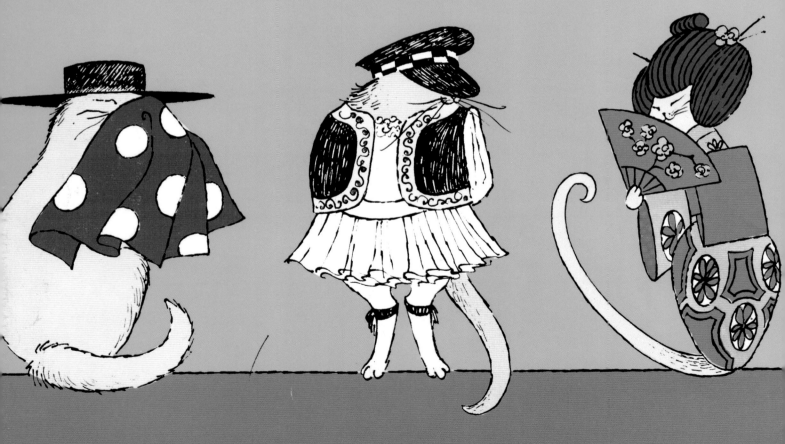

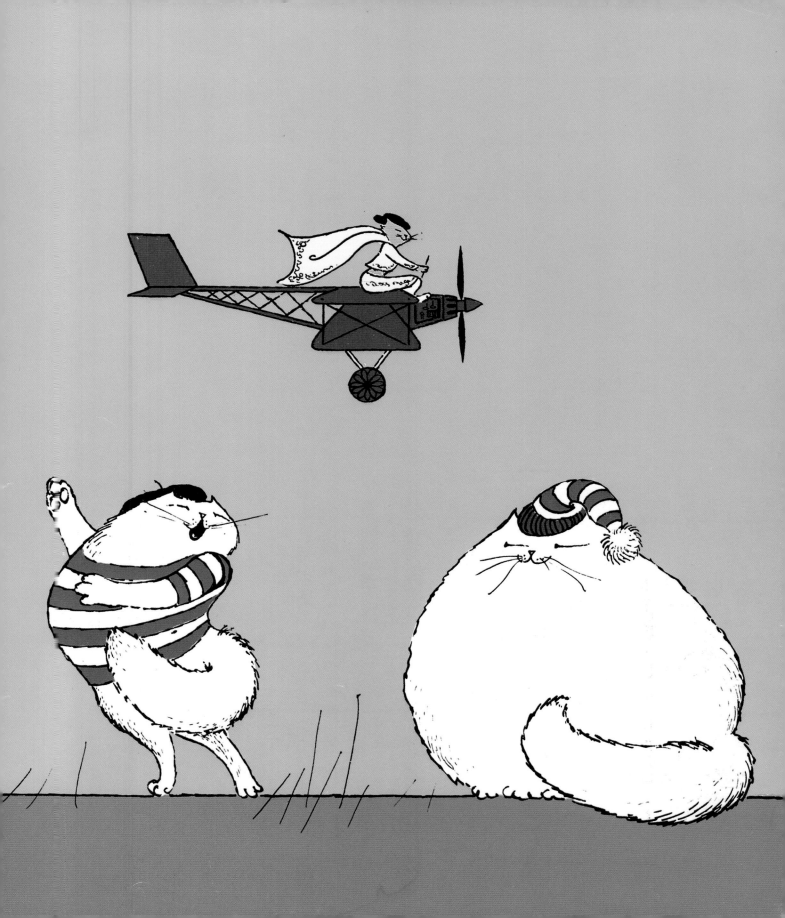

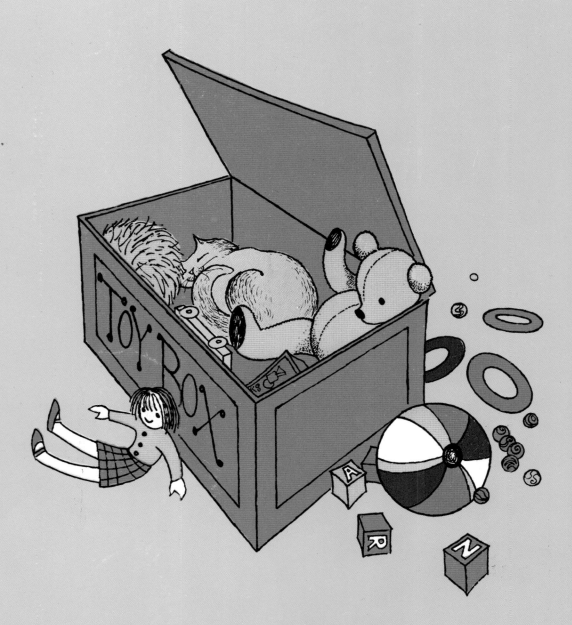

BUT MY CAT LIKES TO HIDE IN BOXES.